# Baby Shower For

________________________________

________________________________

## Date

________________________________

________________________________

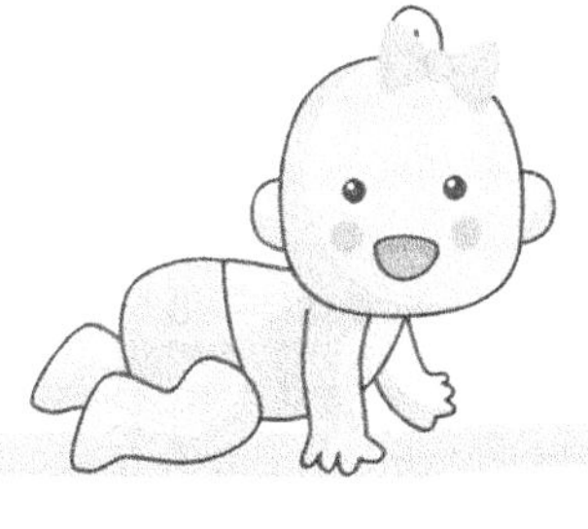
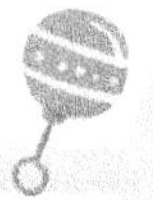

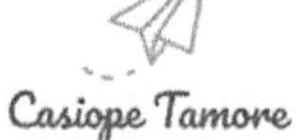

Guest Name

Relationship to Parents

Advice for Parents

Wishes for Baby

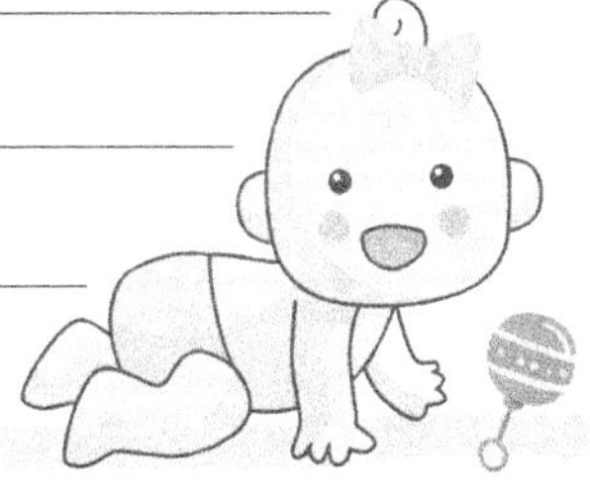

Guest Name

Relationship to Parents

Advice for Parents

Wishes for Baby

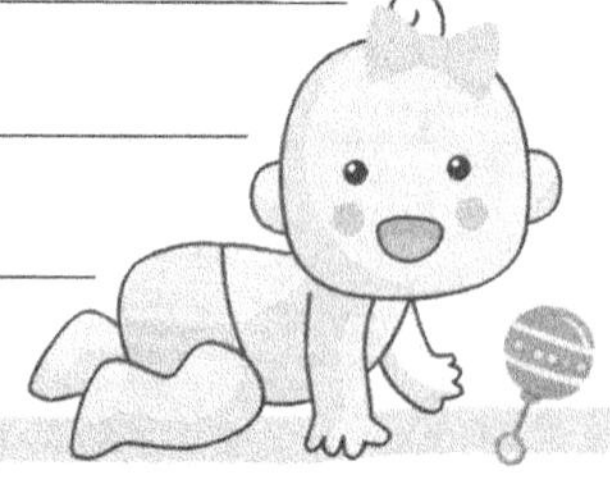

Guest Name

___________________________________________

Relationship to Parents

___________________________________________

Advice for Parents

___________________________________________

___________________________________________

___________________________________________

Wishes for Baby

___________________________________________

___________________________________________

___________________________________________

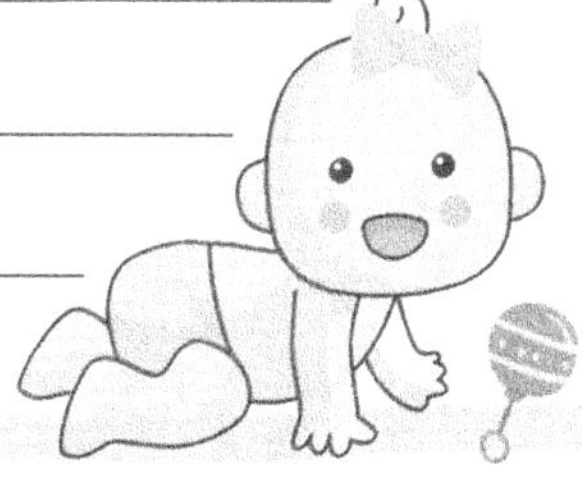

Guest Name

Relationship to Parents

Advice for Parents

Wishes for Baby

Guest Name

Relationship to Parents

Advice for Parents

Wishes for Baby

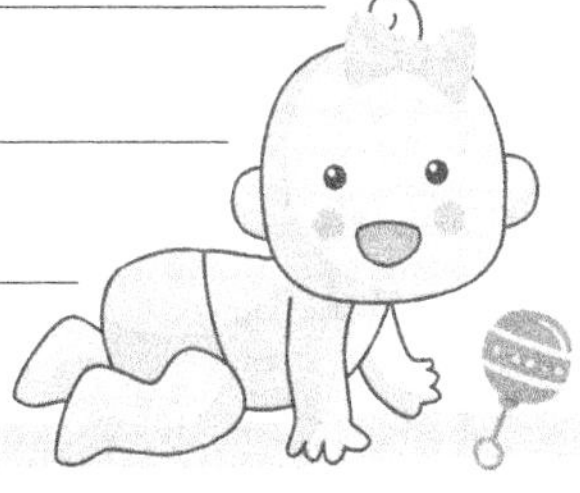

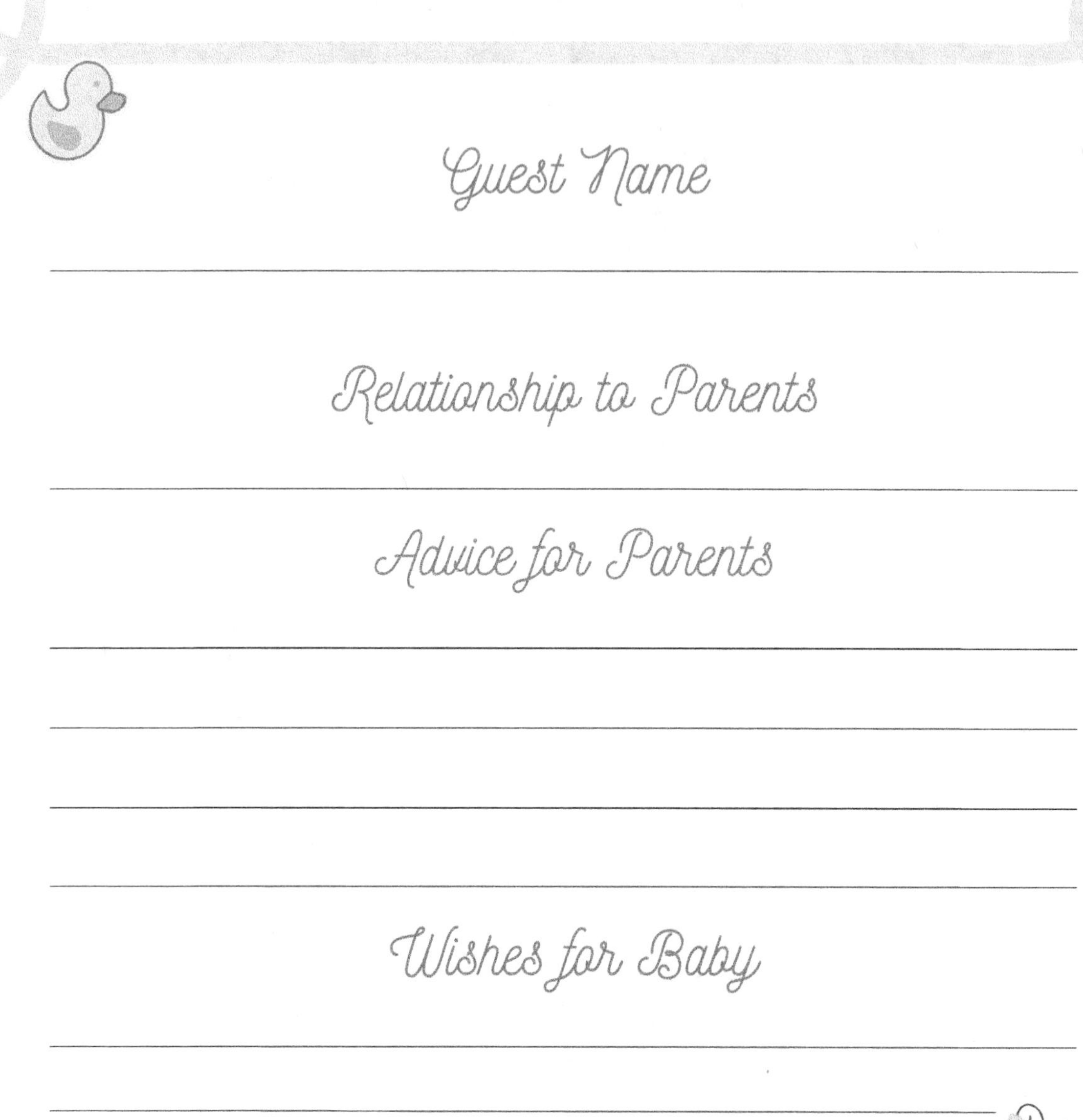

Guest Name
Relationship to Parents
Advice for Parents
Wishes for Baby

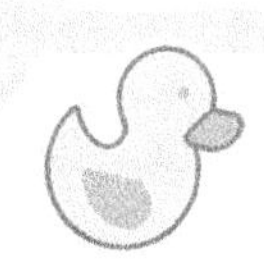

Guest Name

Relationship to Parents

Advice for Parents

Wishes for Baby

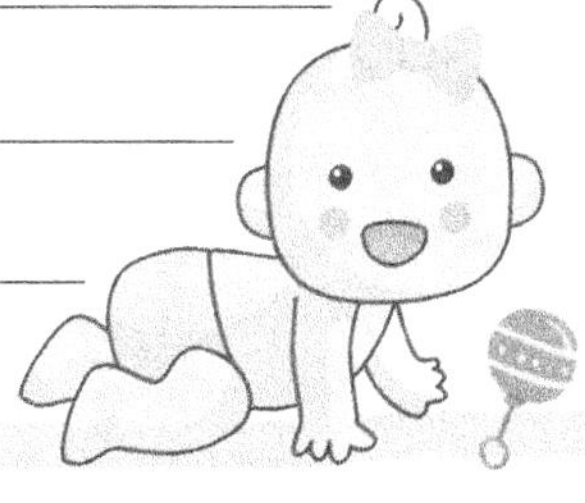

Guest Name

Relationship to Parents

Advice for Parents

Wishes for Baby

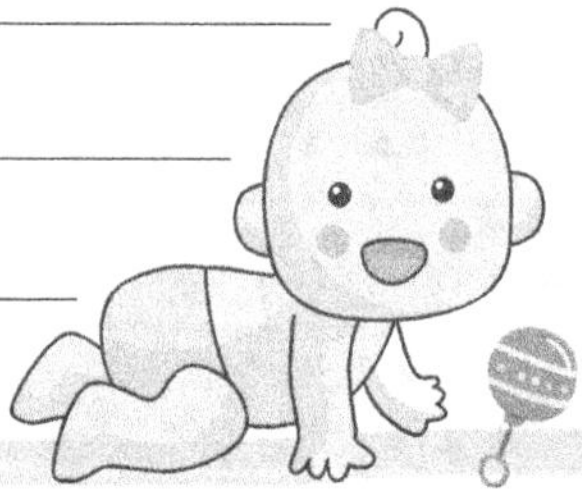

Guest Name

Relationship to Parents

Advice for Parents

Wishes for Baby

Guest Name

_______________________________

Relationship to Parents

_______________________________

Advice for Parents

_______________________________

_______________________________

_______________________________

_______________________________

Wishes for Baby

_______________________________

_______________________________

_______________________________

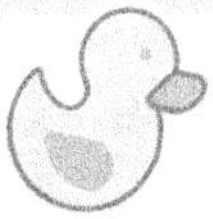

Guest Name

Relationship to Parents

Advice for Parents

Wishes for Baby

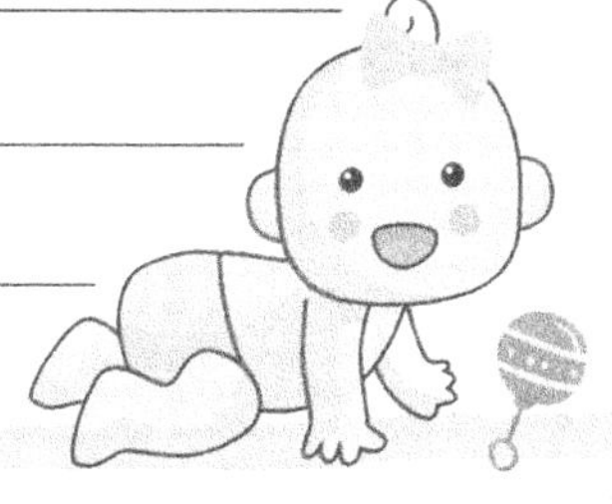

Guest Name

Relationship to Parents

Advice for Parents

Wishes for Baby

Guest Name

Relationship to Parents

Advice for Parents

Wishes for Baby

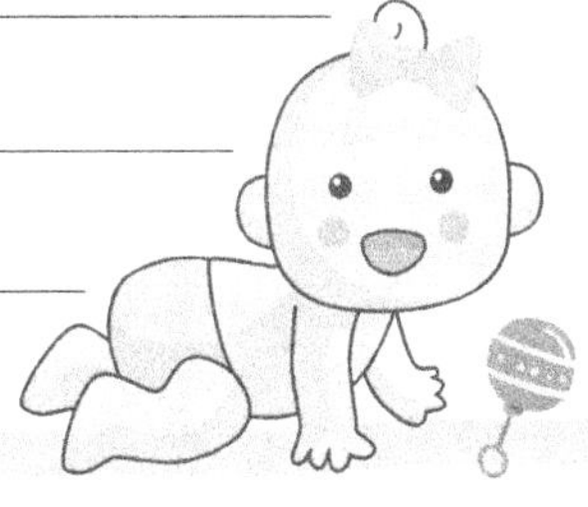

Guest Name

Relationship to Parents

Advice for Parents

Wishes for Baby

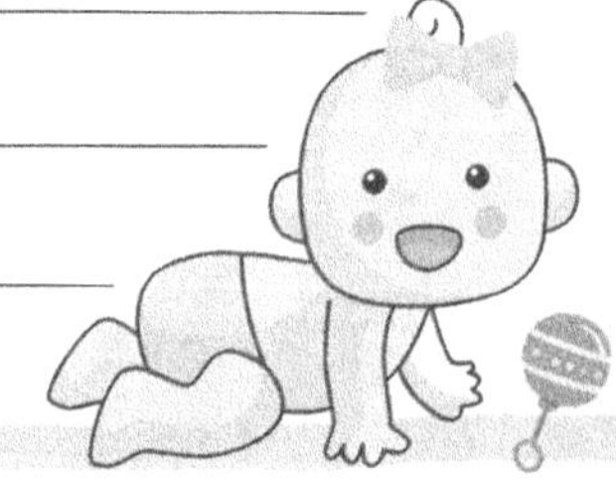

Guest Name

Relationship to Parents

Advice for Parents

Wishes for Baby

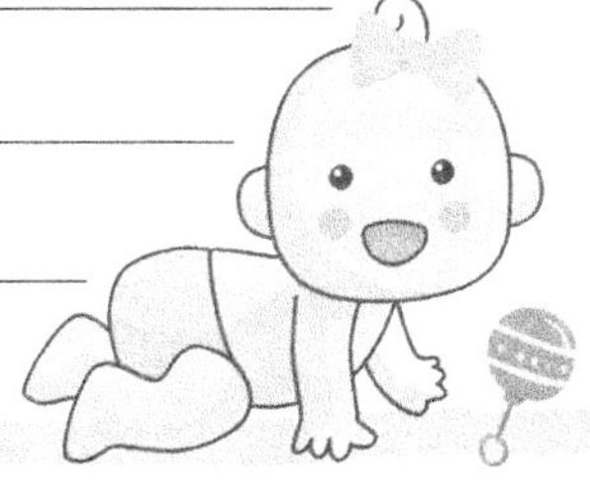

Guest Name

Relationship to Parents

Advice for Parents

Wishes for Baby

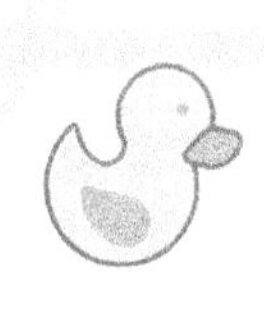

Guest Name

Relationship to Parents

Advice for Parents

Wishes for Baby

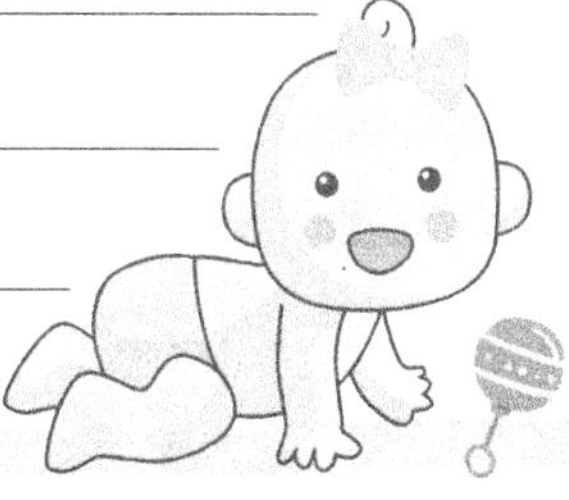

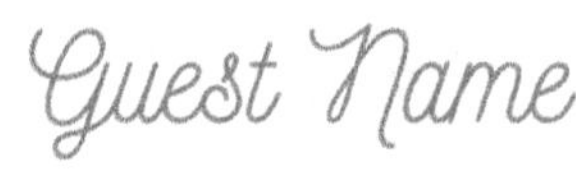

Guest Name

___________________________________

Relationship to Parents

___________________________________

Advice for Parents

___________________________________

___________________________________

___________________________________

___________________________________

Wishes for Baby

___________________________________

___________________________________

___________________________________

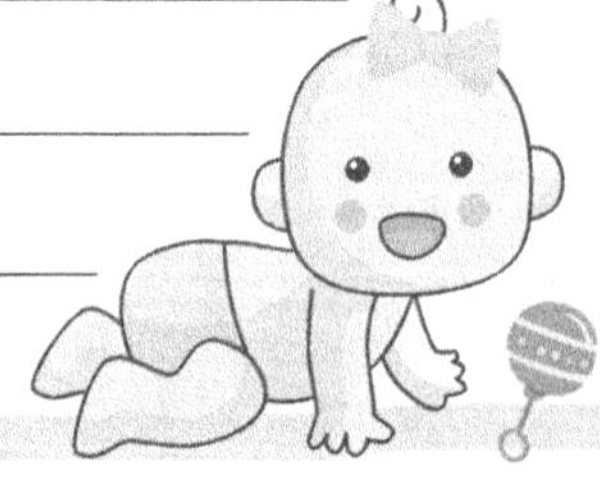

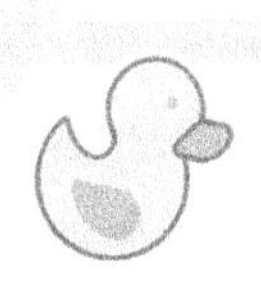

Guest Name

Relationship to Parents

Advice for Parents

Wishes for Baby

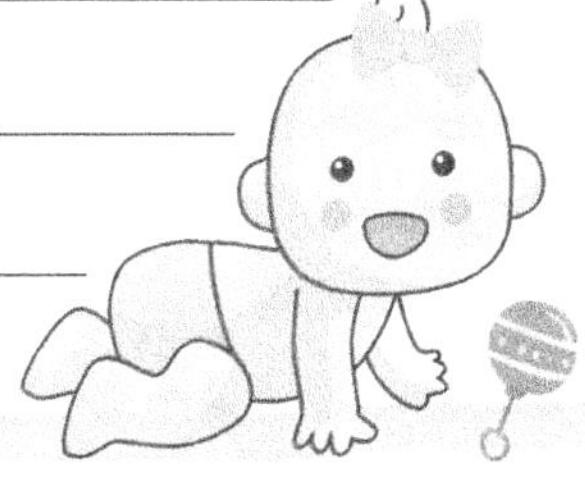

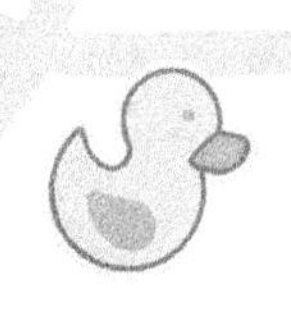

Guest Name

Relationship to Parents

Advice for Parents

Wishes for Baby

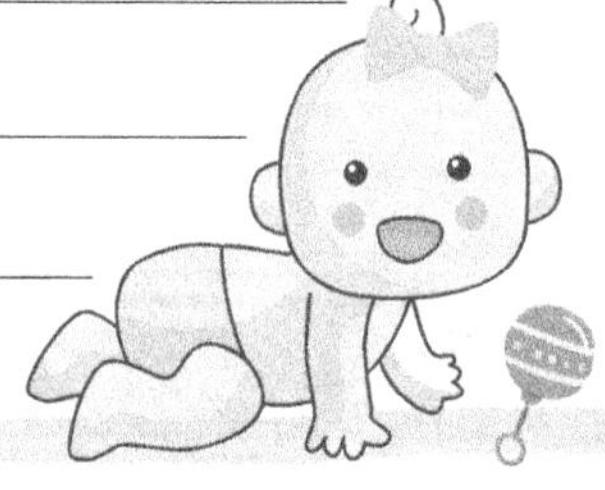

Guest Name

Relationship to Parents

Advice for Parents

Wishes for Baby

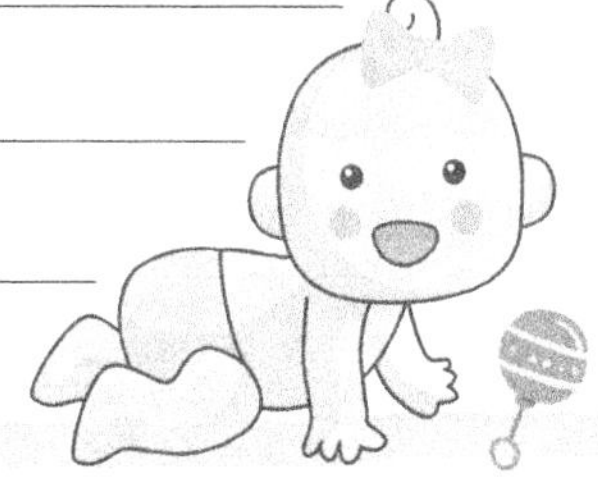

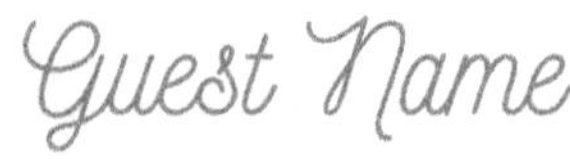

Guest Name

___

Relationship to Parents

___

Advice for Parents

___

___

___

___

Wishes for Baby

___

___

___

___

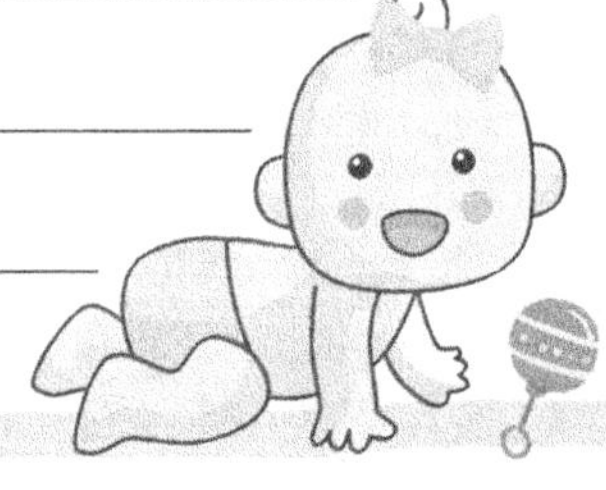

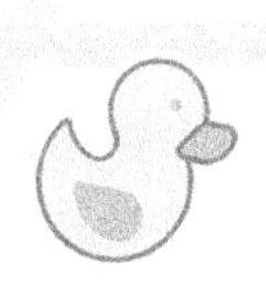

Guest Name

___________________________

Relationship to Parents

___________________________

Advice for Parents

___________________________

___________________________

___________________________

___________________________

Wishes for Baby

___________________________

___________________________

___________________________

___________________________

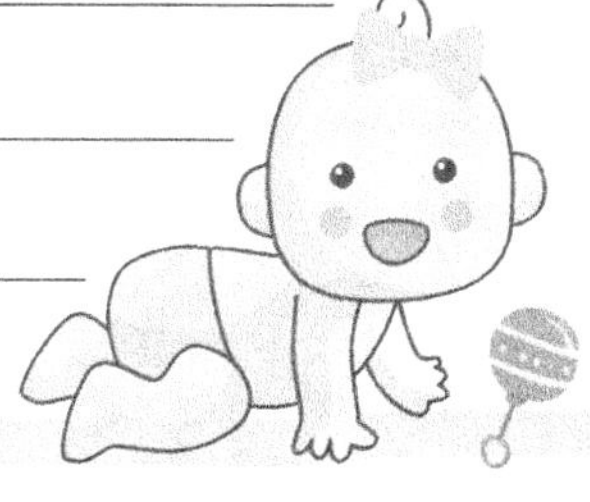

Guest Name

Relationship to Parents

Advice for Parents

Wishes for Baby

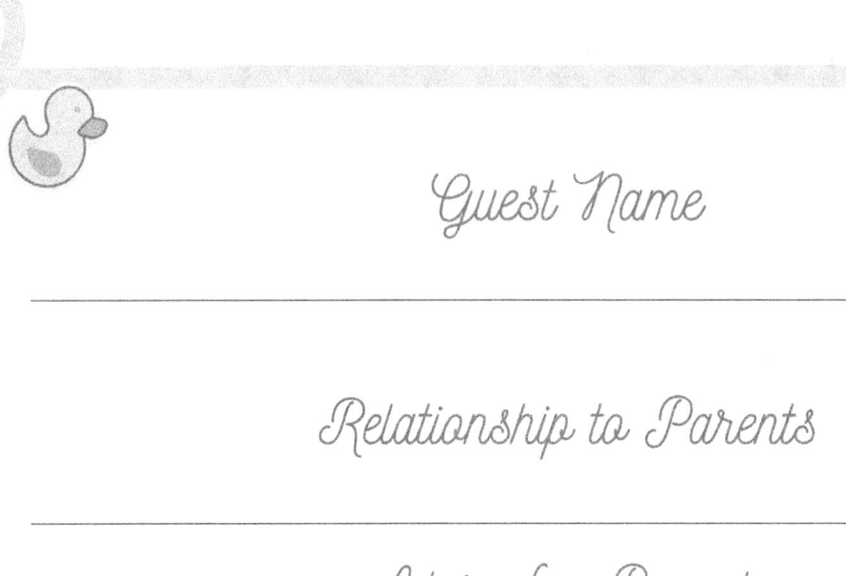

Guest Name

Relationship to Parents

Advice for Parents

Wishes for Baby

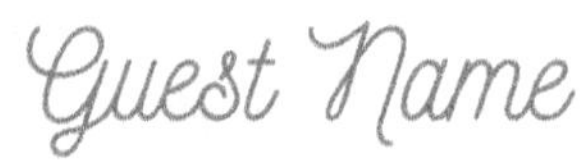

Guest Name

Relationship to Parents

Advice for Parents

Wishes for Baby

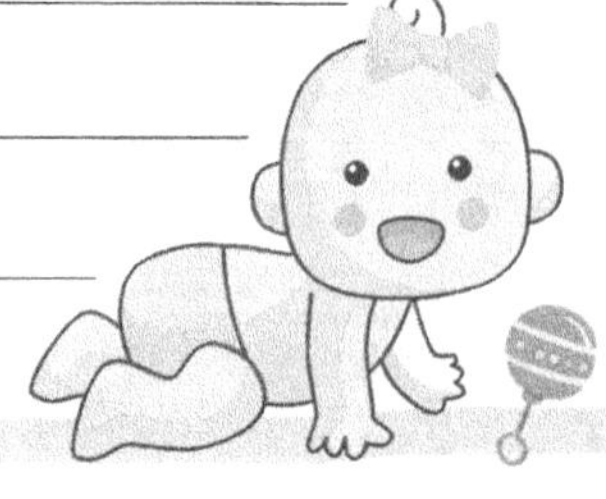

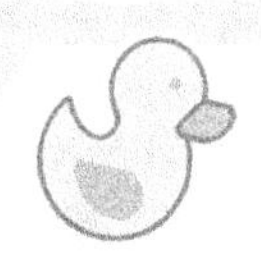

Guest Name

Relationship to Parents

Advice for Parents

Wishes for Baby

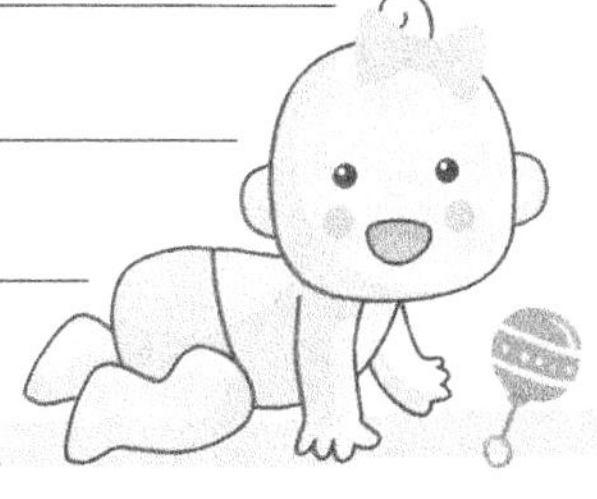

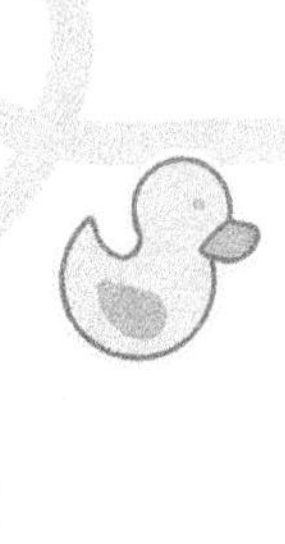

Guest Name

Relationship to Parents

Advice for Parents

Wishes for Baby

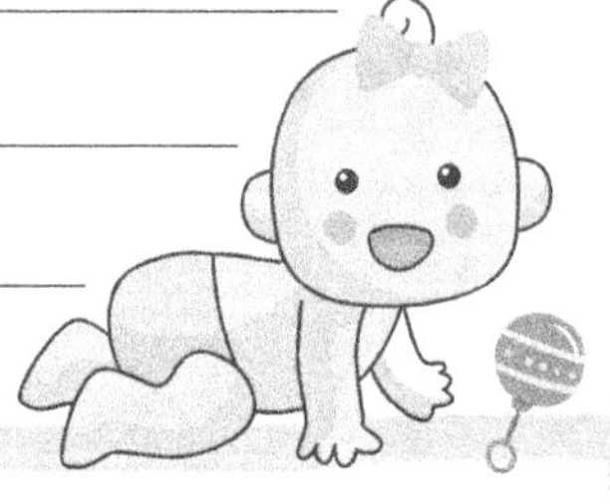

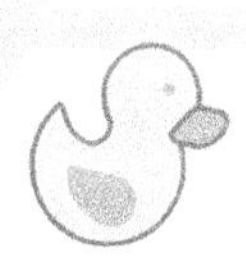

Guest Name

Relationship to Parents

Advice for Parents

Wishes for Baby

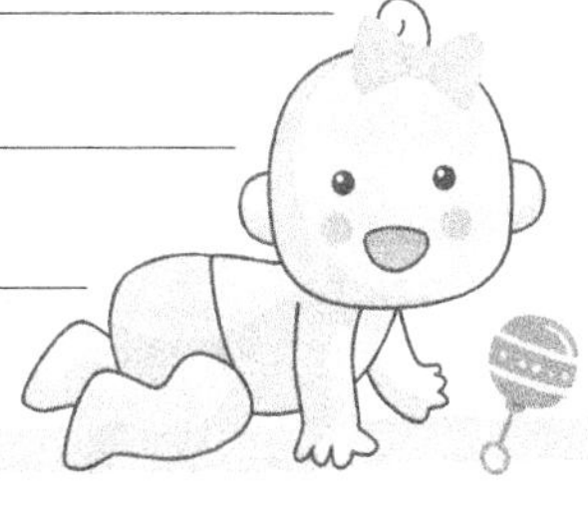

Guest Name

Relationship to Parents

Advice for Parents

Wishes for Baby

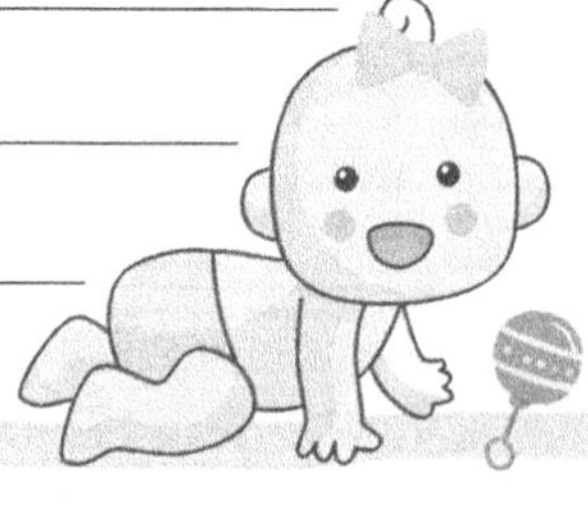

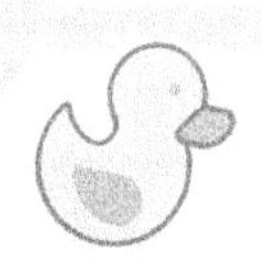

Guest Name

Relationship to Parents

Advice for Parents

Wishes for Baby

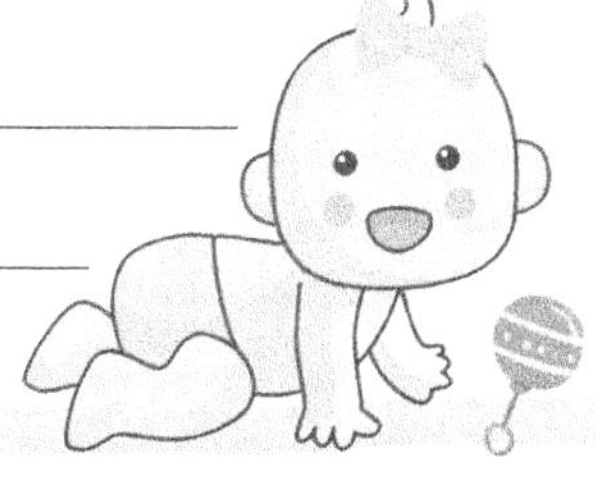

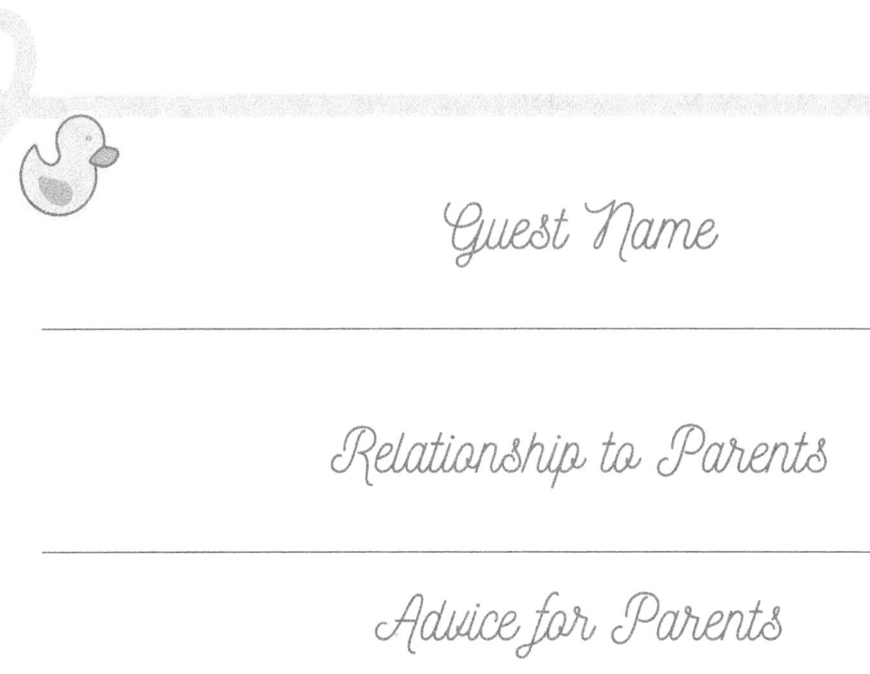

Guest Name

Relationship to Parents

Advice for Parents

Wishes for Baby

Guest Name

Relationship to Parents

Advice for Parents

Wishes for Baby

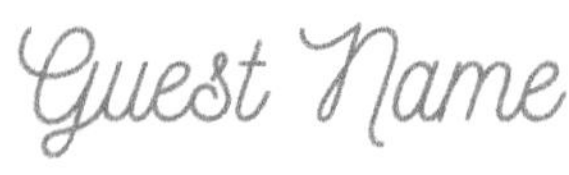

Guest Name

_______________________________

Relationship to Parents

_______________________________

Advice for Parents

_______________________________

_______________________________

_______________________________

_______________________________

Wishes for Baby

_______________________________

_______________________________

_______________________________

_______________________________

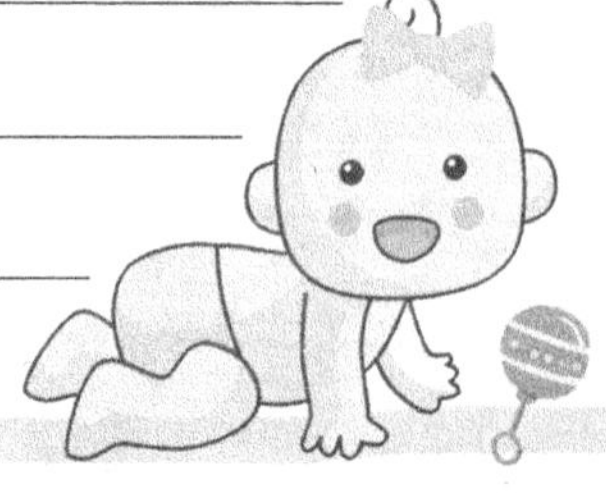

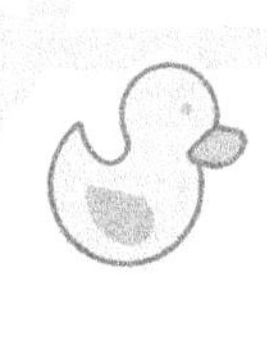

Guest Name

_______________________________________________

Relationship to Parents

_______________________________________________

Advice for Parents

_______________________________________________

_______________________________________________

_______________________________________________

Wishes for Baby

_______________________________________________

_______________________________________________

_______________________________________________

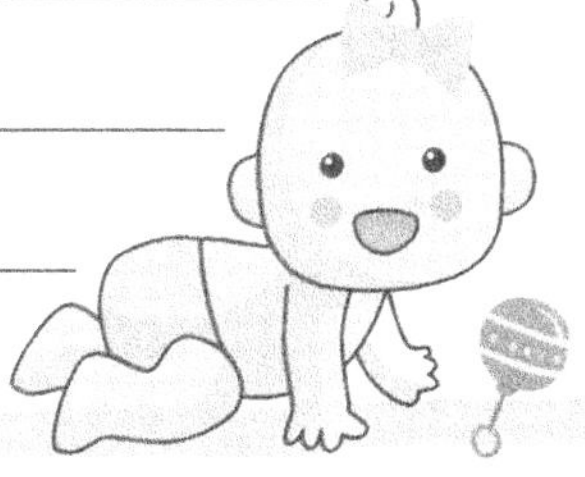

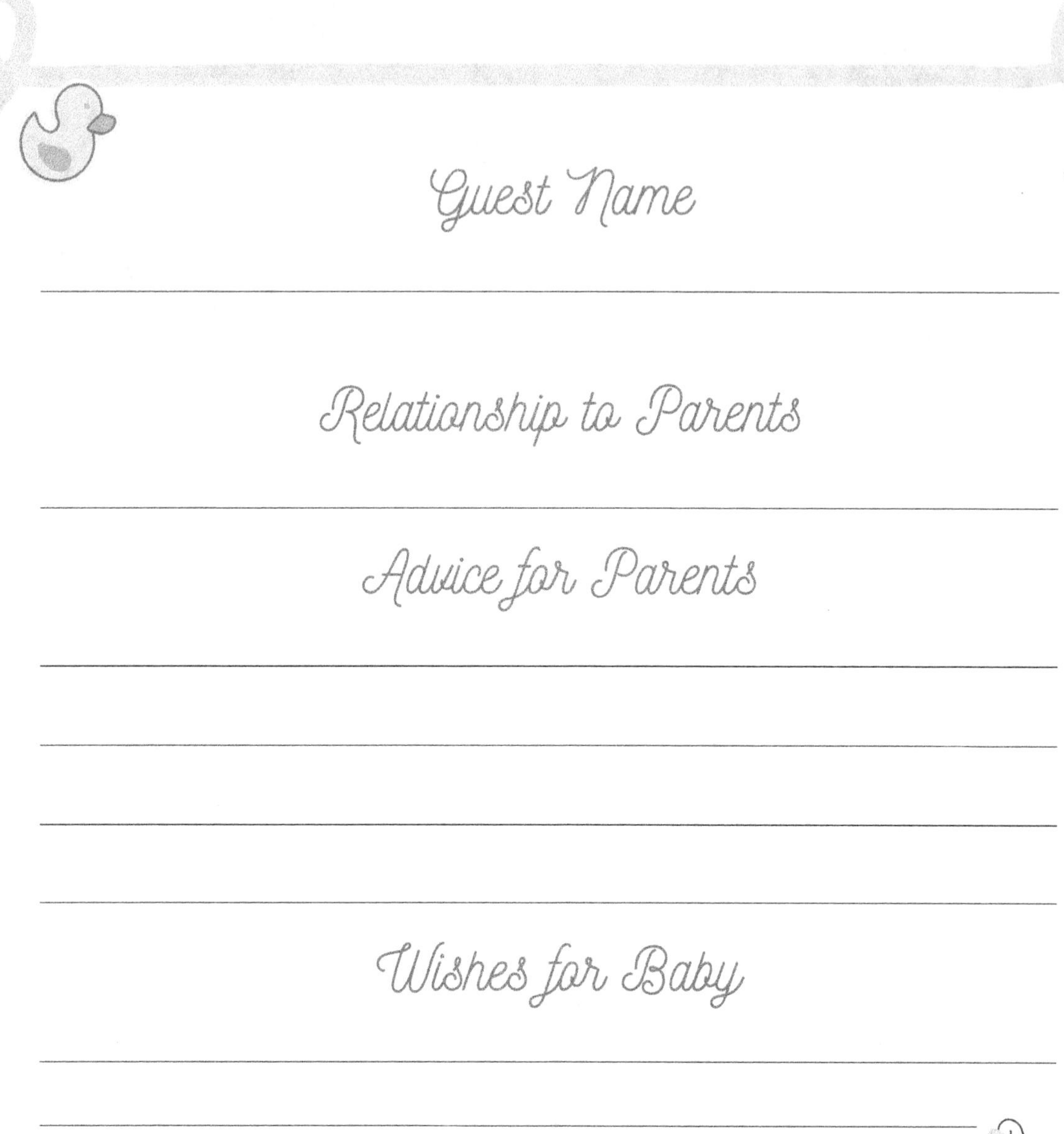

Guest Name

_______________________________

Relationship to Parents

_______________________________

Advice for Parents

_______________________________

_______________________________

_______________________________

_______________________________

Wishes for Baby

_______________________________

_______________________________

_______________________________

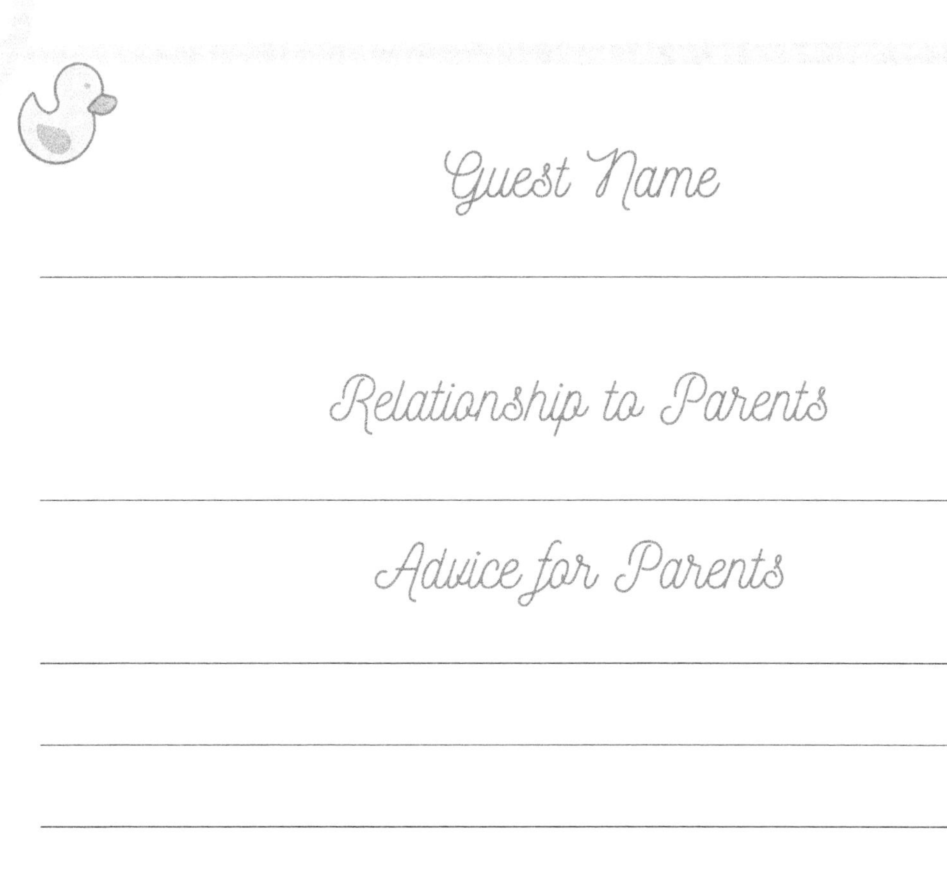

Guest Name

Relationship to Parents

Advice for Parents

Wishes for Baby

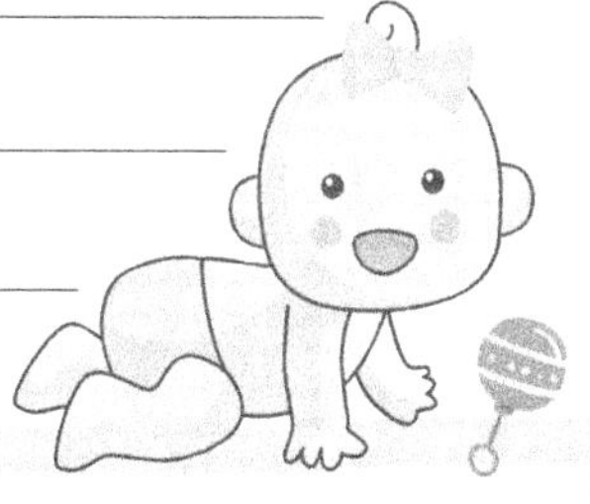

Guest Name

_______________________________________________

Relationship to Parents

_______________________________________________

Advice for Parents

_______________________________________________

_______________________________________________

_______________________________________________

_______________________________________________

Wishes for Baby

_______________________________________________

_______________________________________________

_______________________________________________

_______________________________________________

Guest Name

Relationship to Parents

Advice for Parents

Wishes for Baby

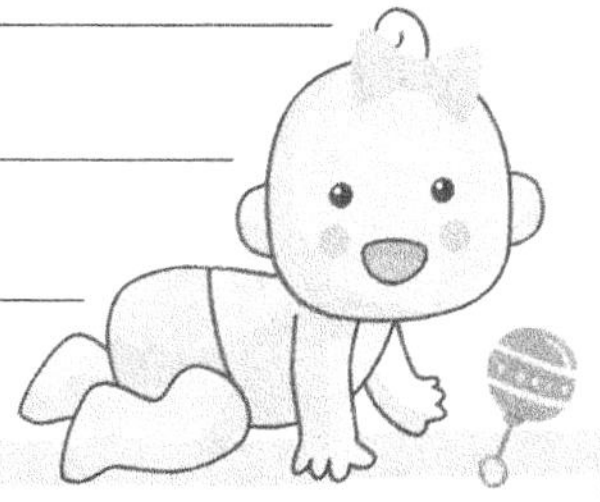

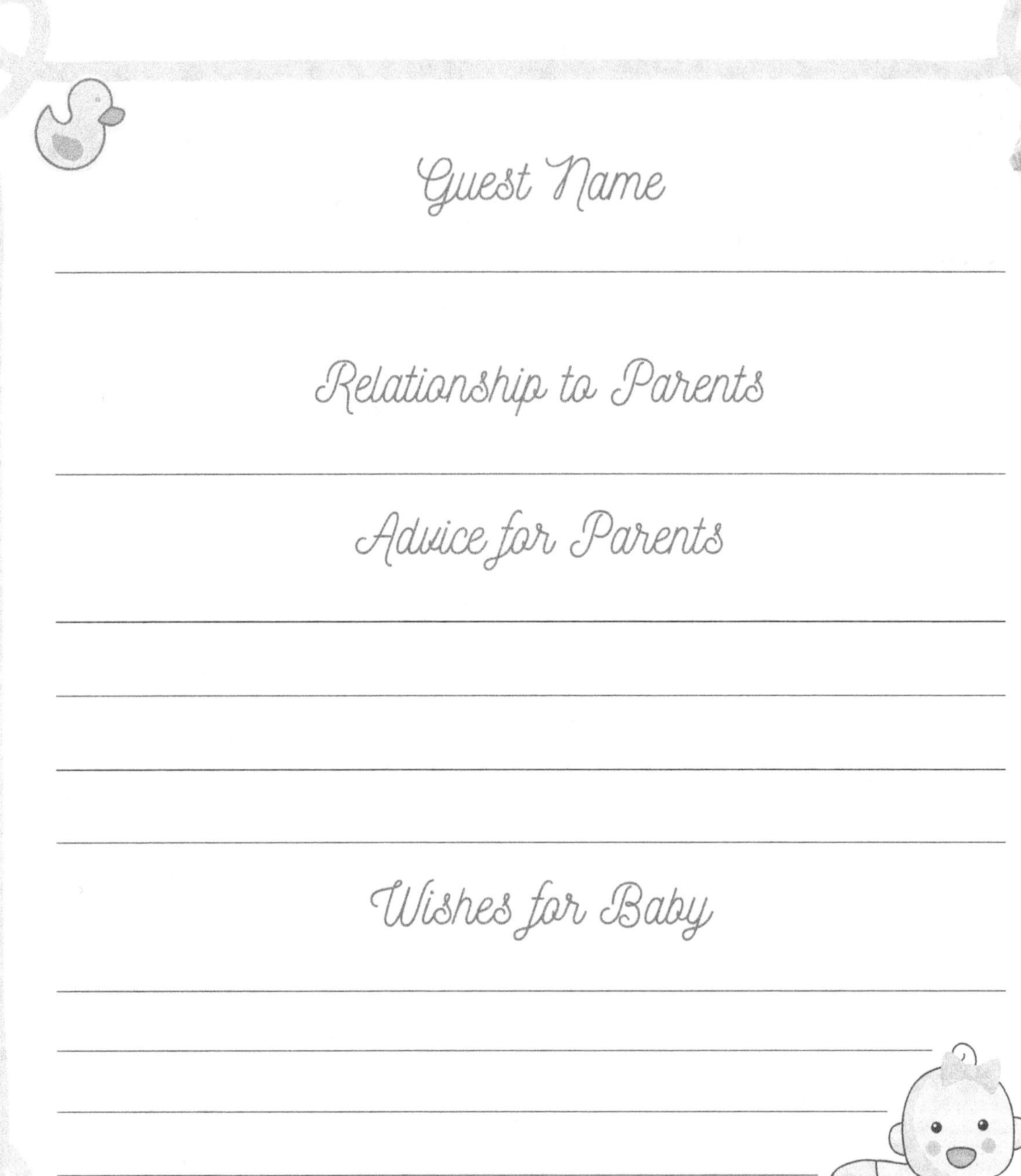

Guest Name

Relationship to Parents

Advice for Parents

Wishes for Baby

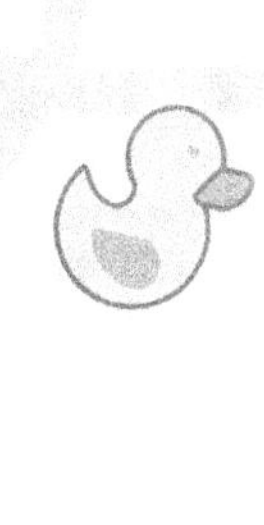

Guest Name

Relationship to Parents

Advice for Parents

Wishes for Baby

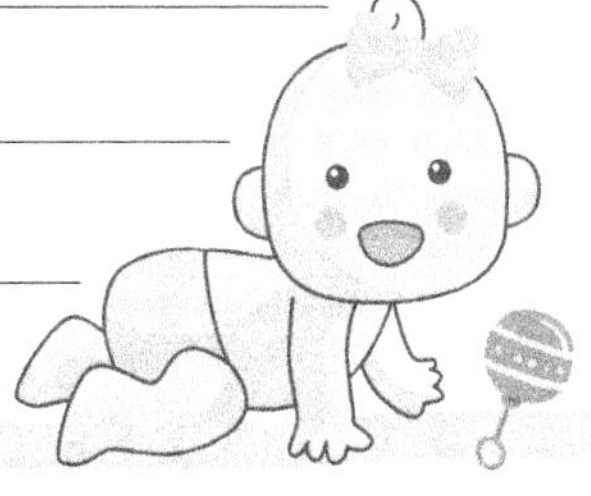

Guest Name

Relationship to Parents

Advice for Parents

Wishes for Baby

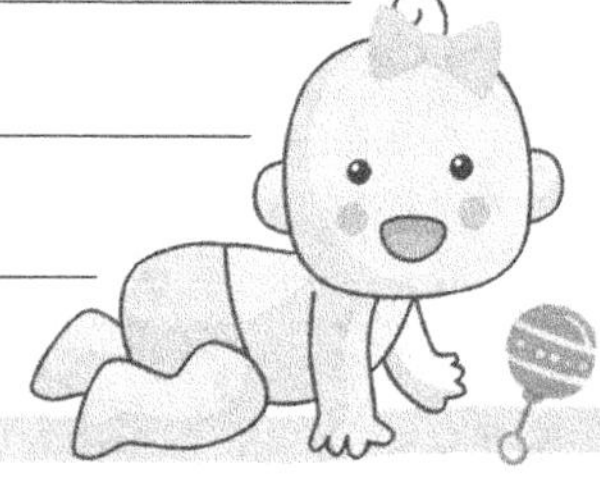

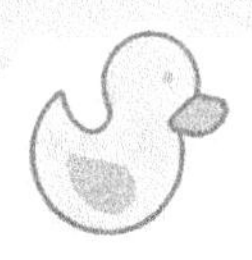

Guest Name

Relationship to Parents

Advice for Parents

Wishes for Baby

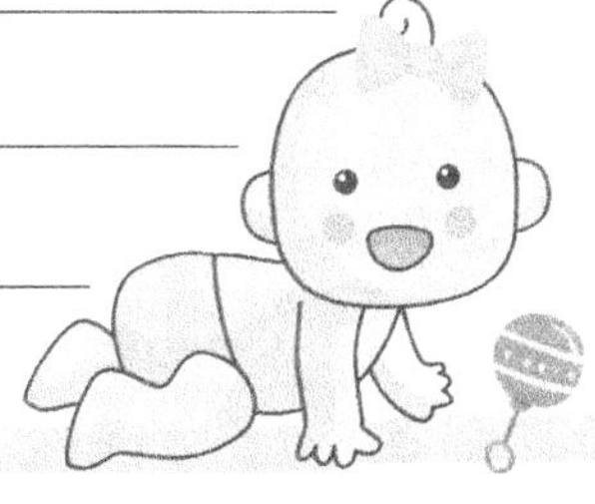

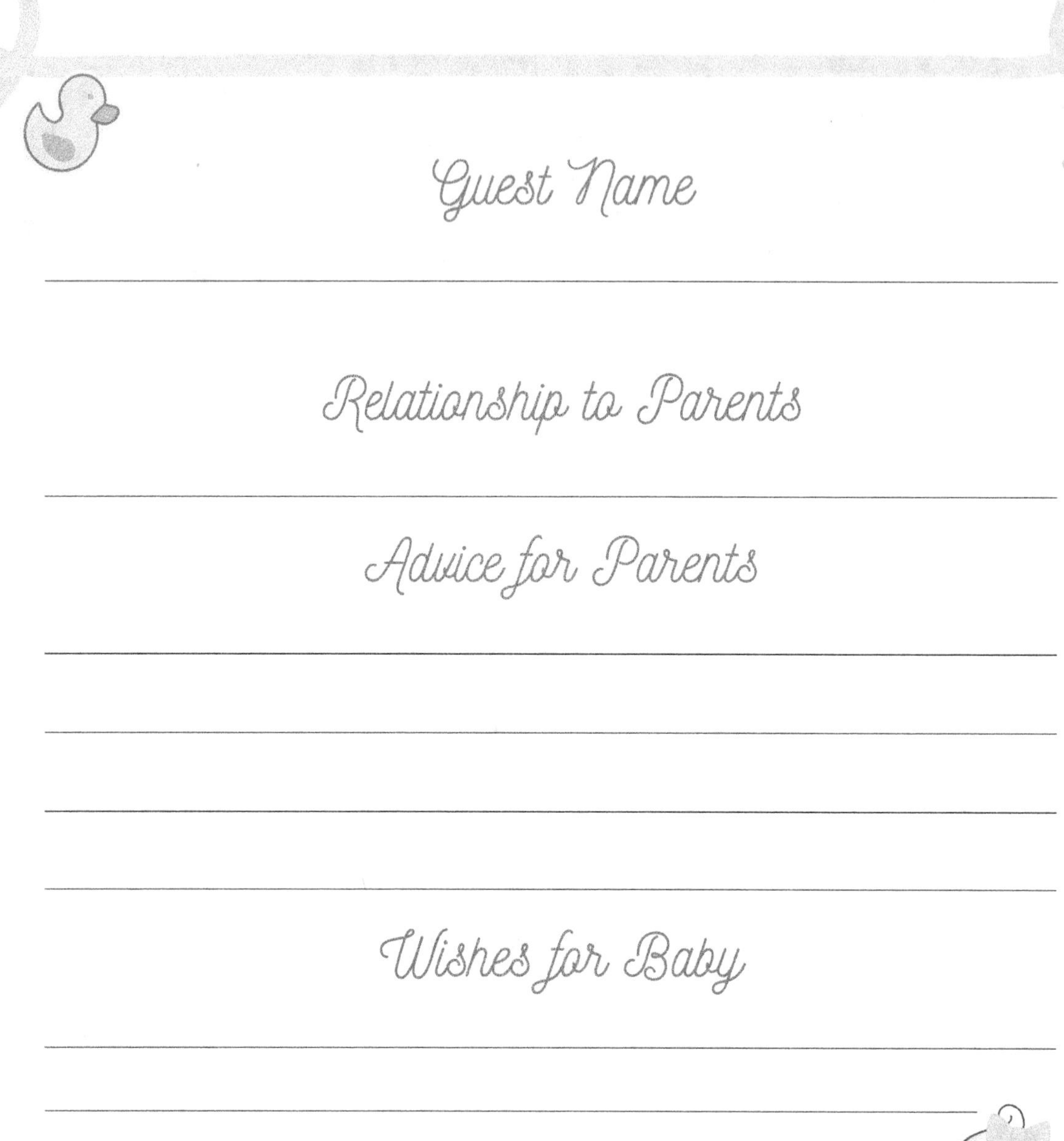

Guest Name

Relationship to Parents

Advice for Parents

Wishes for Baby

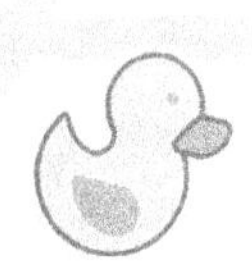

Guest Name

_______________________________________________

Relationship to Parents

_______________________________________________

Advice for Parents

_______________________________________________

_______________________________________________

_______________________________________________

Wishes for Baby

_______________________________________________

_______________________________________________

_______________________________________________

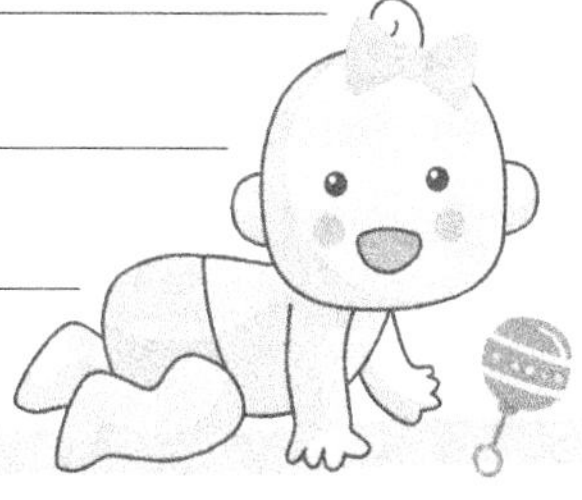

Guest Name

Relationship to Parents

Advice for Parents

Wishes for Baby

Guest Name

Relationship to Parents

Advice for Parents

Wishes for Baby

Guest Name

Relationship to Parents

Advice for Parents

Wishes for Baby

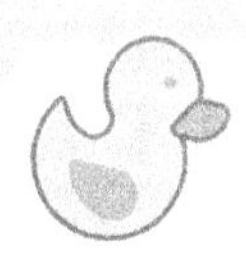

Guest Name

Relationship to Parents

Advice for Parents

Wishes for Baby

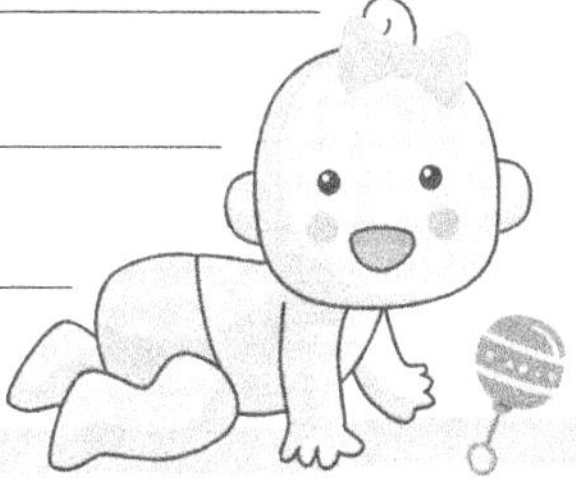

Guest Name

Relationship to Parents

Advice for Parents

Wishes for Baby

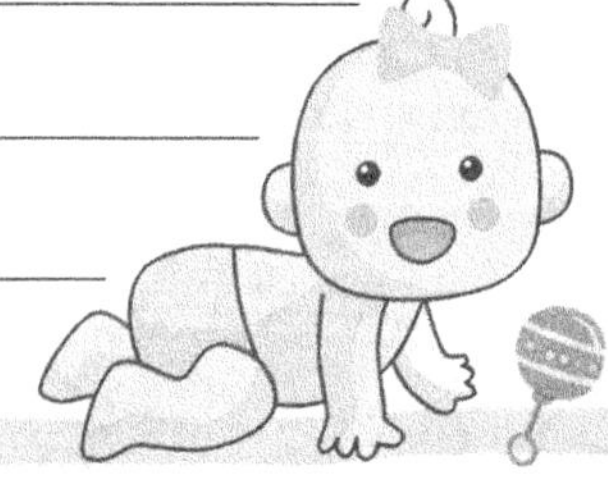

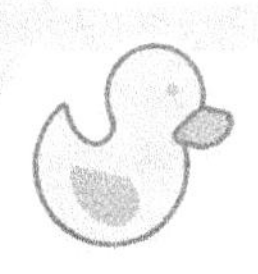

*Guest Name*

*Relationship to Parents*

*Advice for Parents*

*Wishes for Baby*

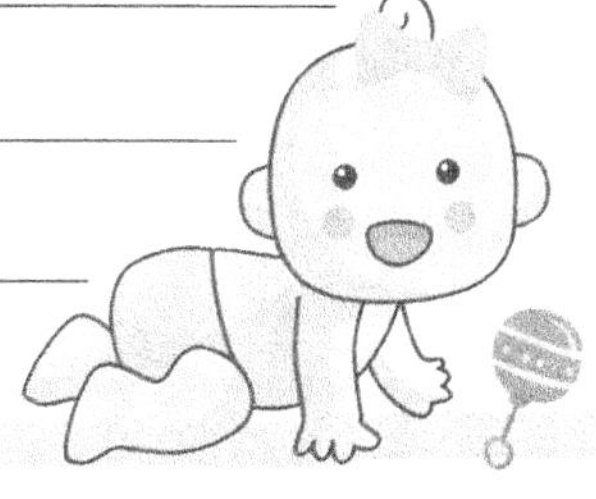

Guest Name

Relationship to Parents

Advice for Parents

Wishes for Baby

Guest Name

Relationship to Parents

Advice for Parents

Wishes for Baby

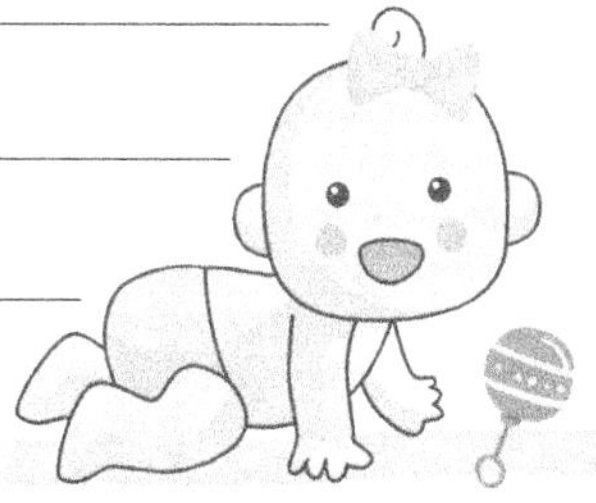

Guest Name

Relationship to Parents

Advice for Parents

Wishes for Baby

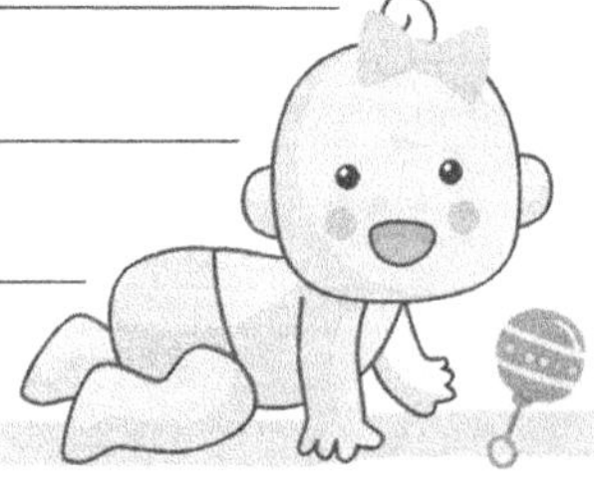

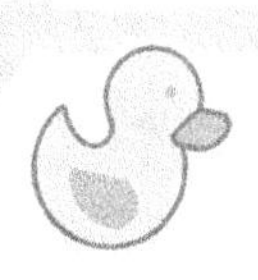

Guest Name

Relationship to Parents

Advice for Parents

Wishes for Baby

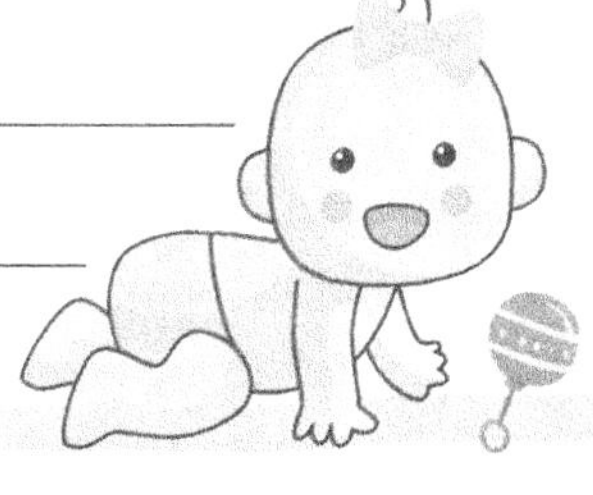

Guest Name

Relationship to Parents

Advice for Parents

Wishes for Baby

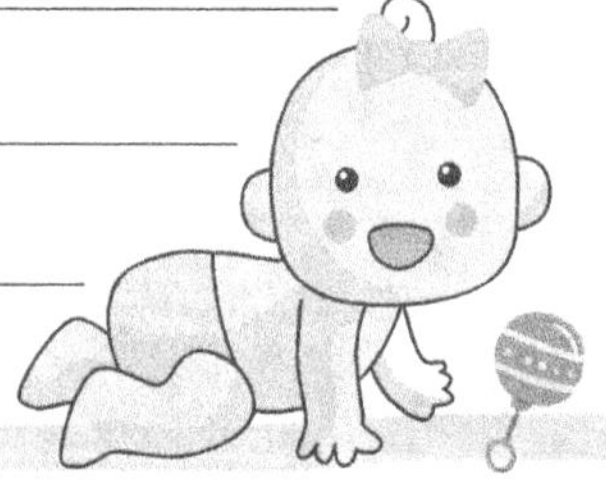

Guest Name

Relationship to Parents

Advice for Parents

Wishes for Baby

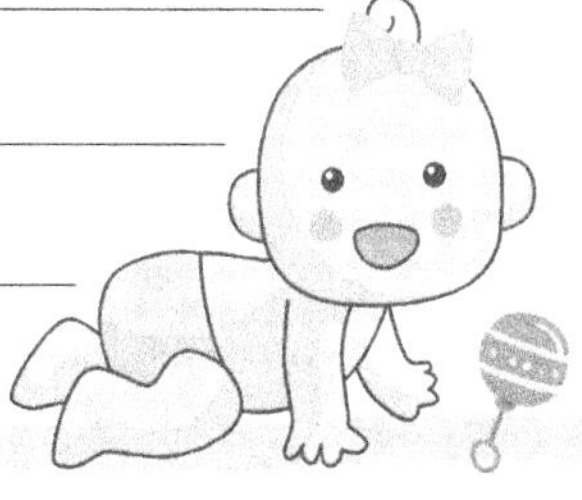

Guest Name

Relationship to Parents

Advice for Parents

Wishes for Baby

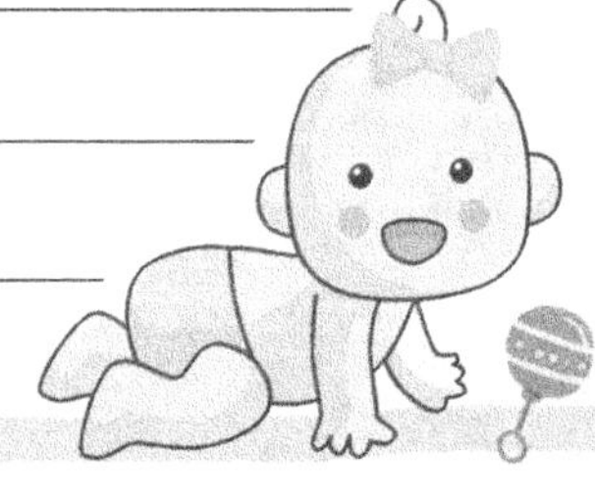

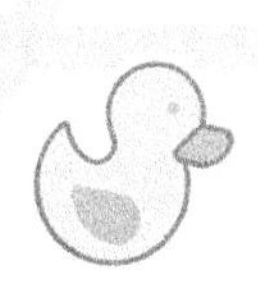

Guest Name

Relationship to Parents

Advice for Parents

Wishes for Baby

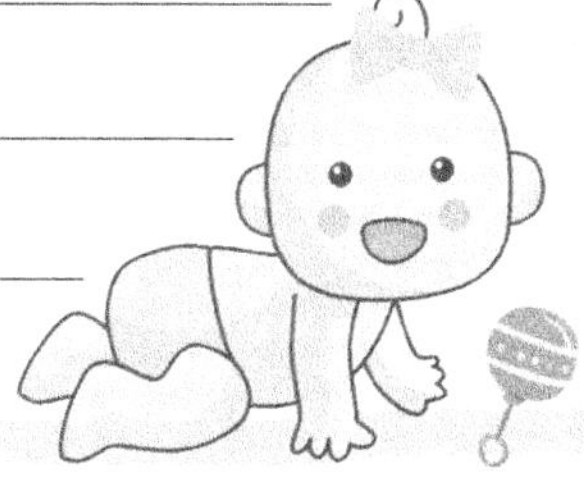

# Guest Name

## Relationship to Parents

## Advice for Parents

## Wishes for Baby

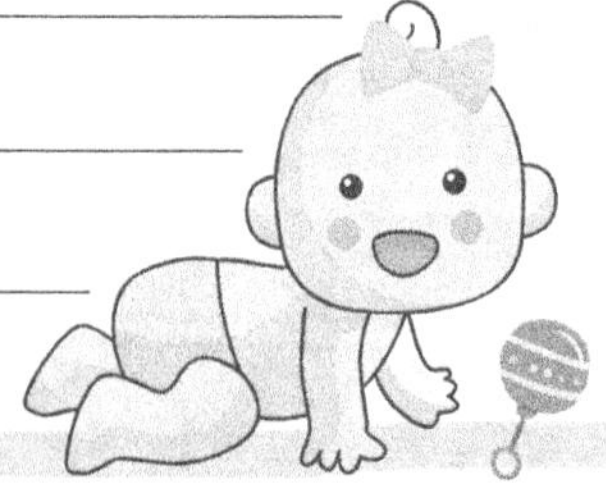

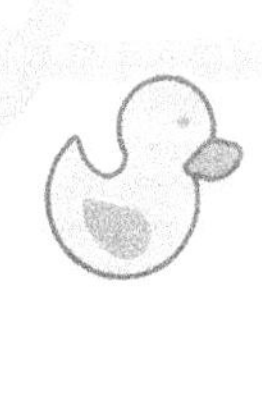

Guest Name

Relationship to Parents

Advice for Parents

Wishes for Baby

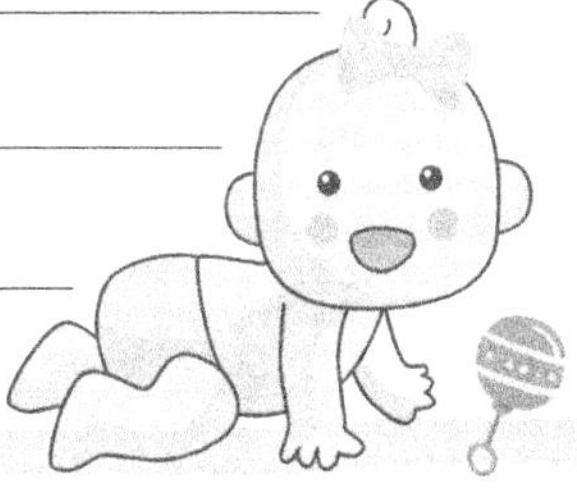

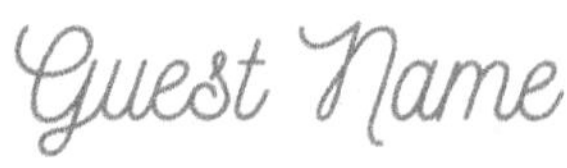

Guest Name

_______________________________

Relationship to Parents

_______________________________

Advice for Parents

_______________________________

_______________________________

_______________________________

_______________________________

Wishes for Baby

_______________________________

_______________________________

_______________________________

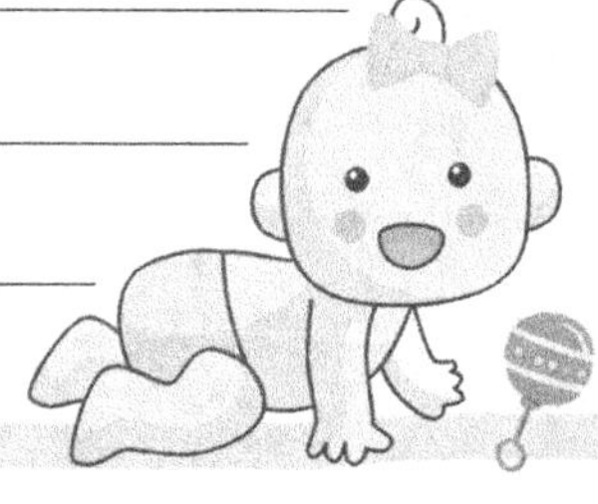

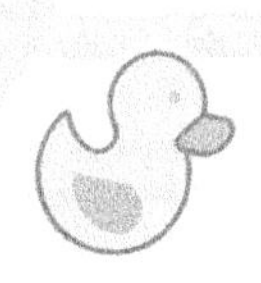

Guest Name

_______________________________________

Relationship to Parents

_______________________________________

Advice for Parents

_______________________________________

_______________________________________

_______________________________________

Wishes for Baby

_______________________________________

_______________________________________

_______________________________________

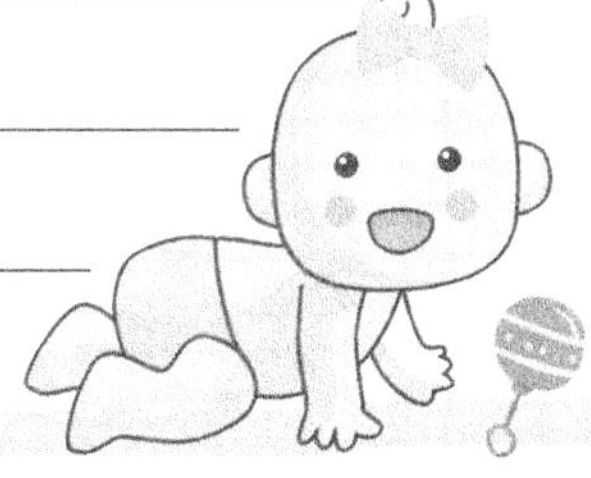

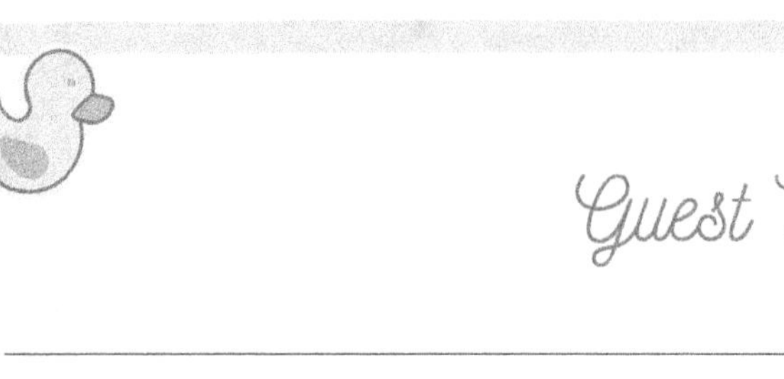

Guest Name

_______________________________________

Relationship to Parents

_______________________________________

Advice for Parents

_______________________________________

_______________________________________

_______________________________________

Wishes for Baby

_______________________________________

_______________________________________

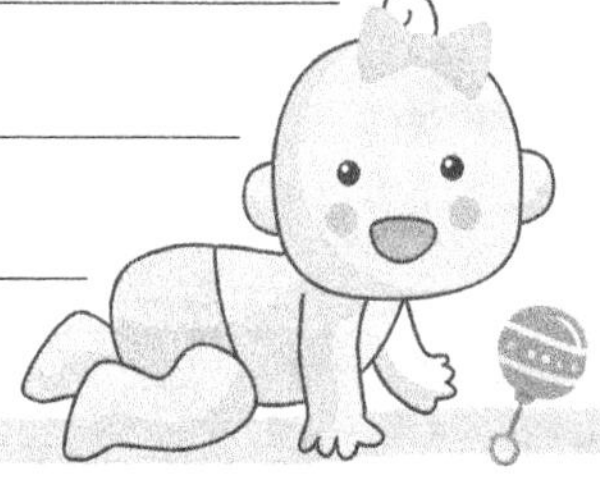

_______________________________________

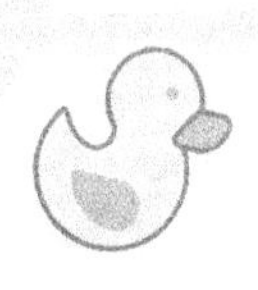

Guest Name

Relationship to Parents

Advice for Parents

Wishes for Baby

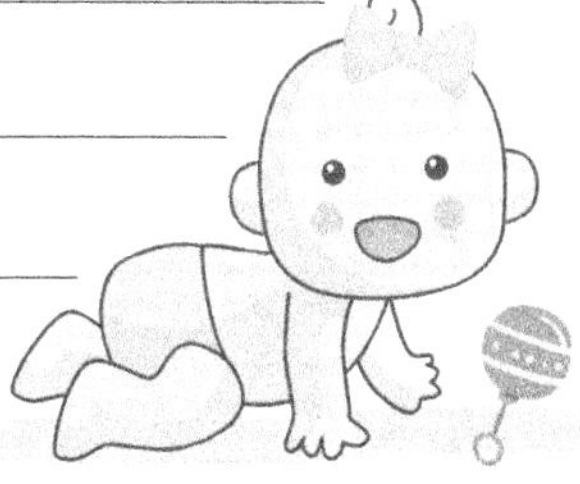

Guest Name

Relationship to Parents

Advice for Parents

Wishes for Baby

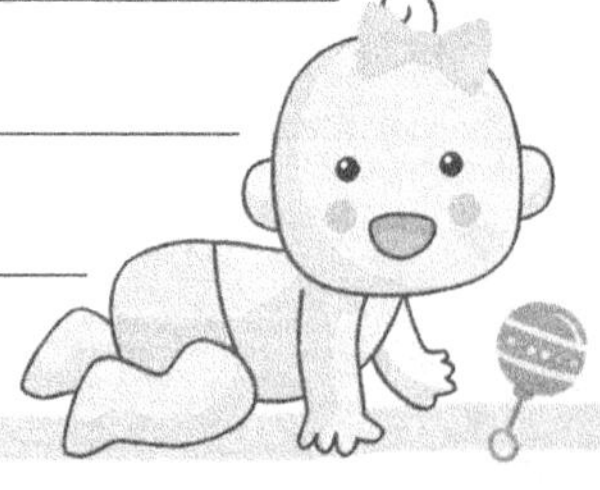

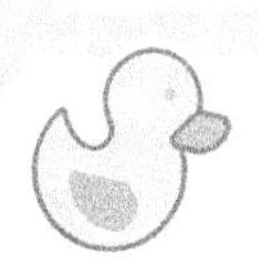

Guest Name

Relationship to Parents

Advice for Parents

Wishes for Baby

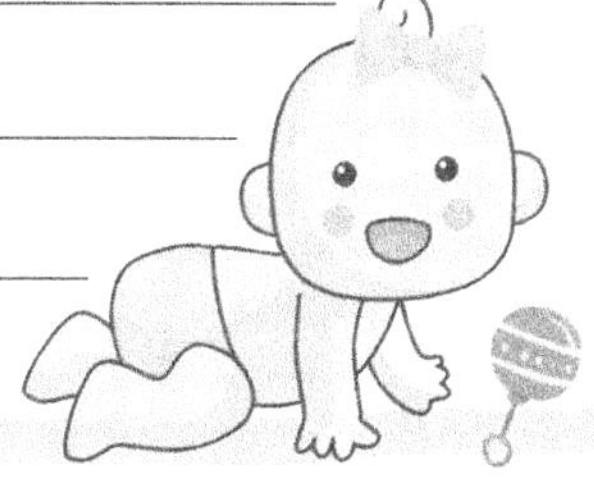

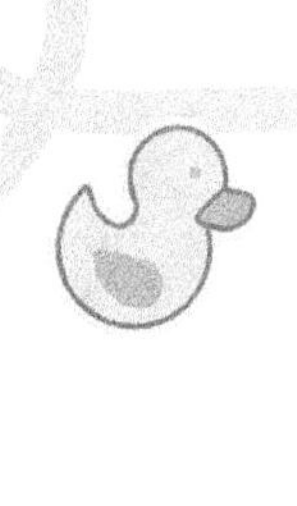

Guest Name

Relationship to Parents

Advice for Parents

Wishes for Baby

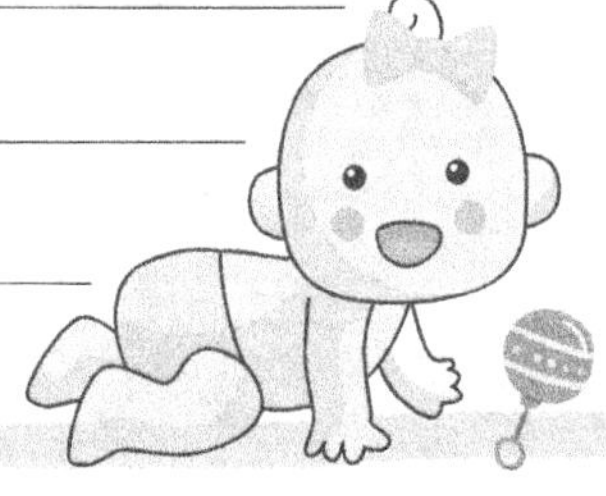

Guest Name

Relationship to Parents

Advice for Parents

Wishes for Baby

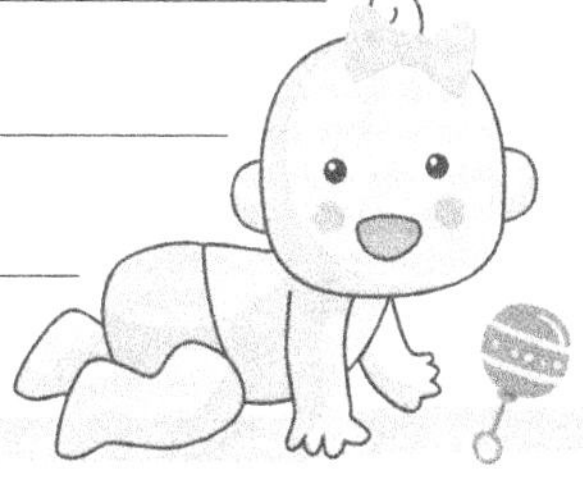

Guest Name

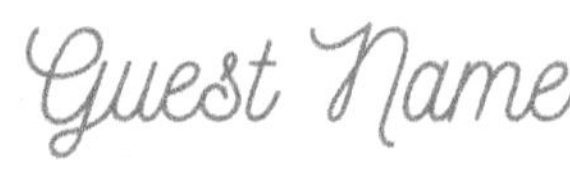

Relationship to Parents

Advice for Parents

Wishes for Baby

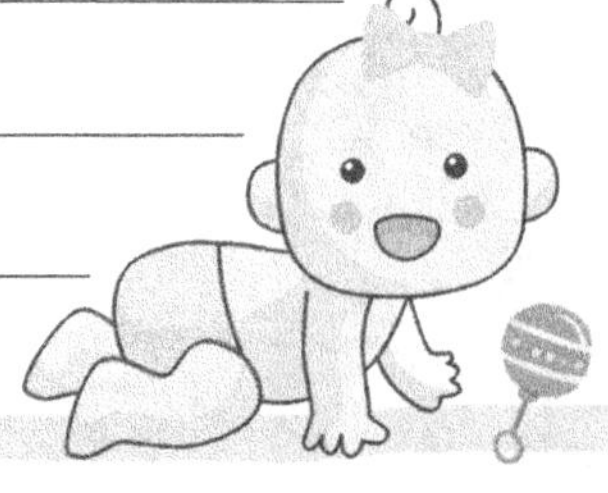

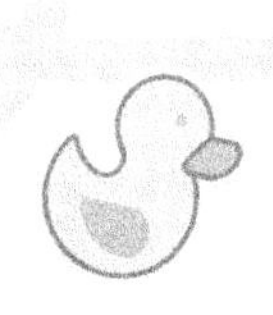

Guest Name

Relationship to Parents

Advice for Parents

Wishes for Baby

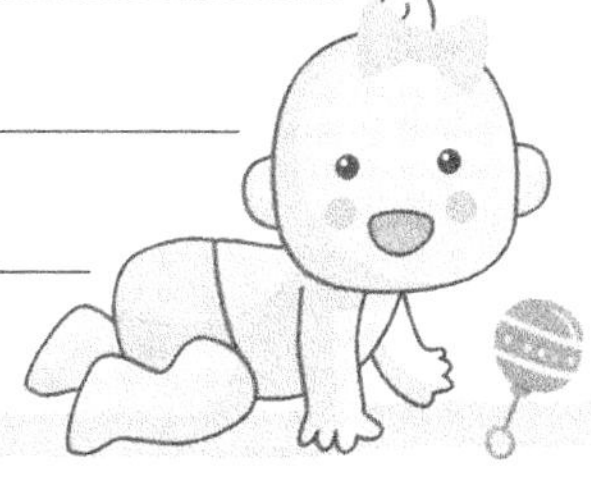

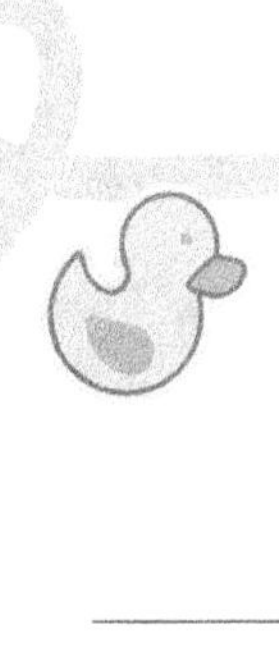

Guest Name

_______________________________________________

Relationship to Parents

_______________________________________________

Advice for Parents

_______________________________________________

_______________________________________________

_______________________________________________

_______________________________________________

Wishes for Baby

_______________________________________________

_______________________________________________

_______________________________________________

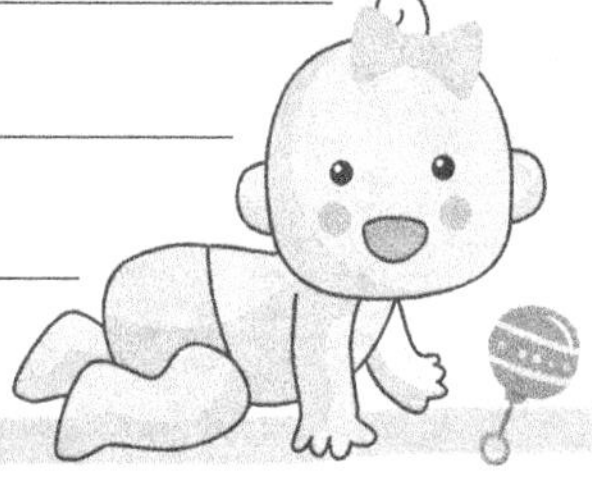

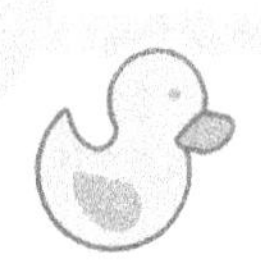

Guest Name

Relationship to Parents

Advice for Parents

Wishes for Baby

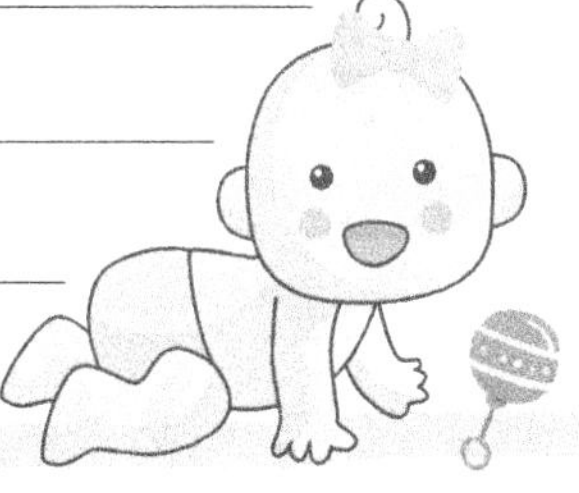

Guest Name

Relationship to Parents

Advice for Parents

Wishes for Baby

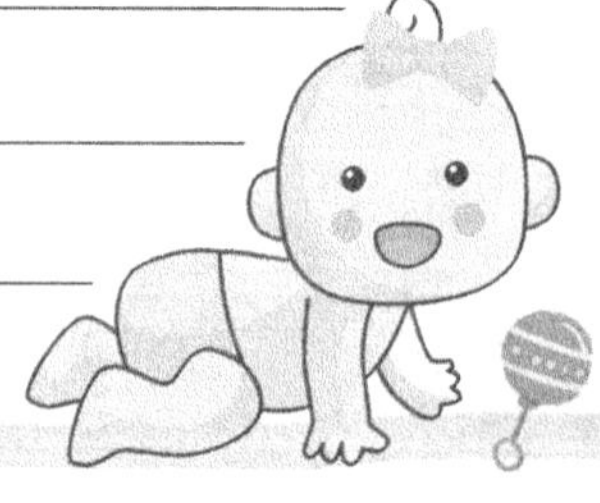

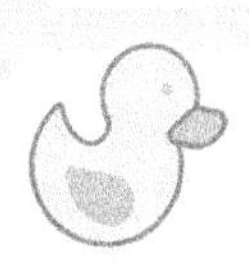

Guest Name

Relationship to Parents

Advice for Parents

Wishes for Baby

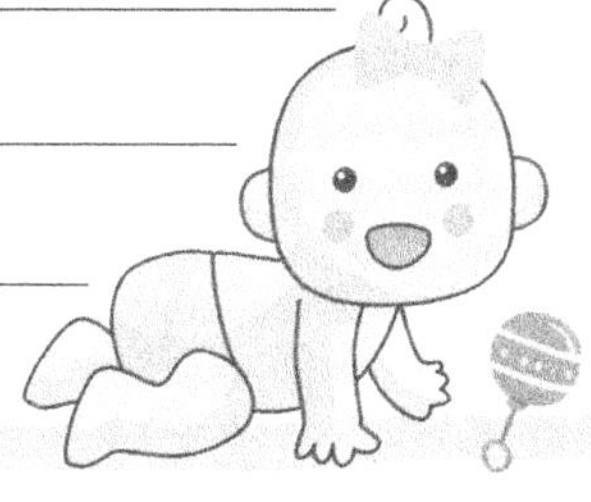

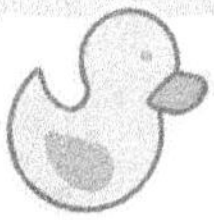

Guest Name

_______________________________________________

Relationship to Parents

_______________________________________________

Advice for Parents

_______________________________________________

_______________________________________________

_______________________________________________

_______________________________________________

Wishes for Baby

_______________________________________________

_______________________________________________

_______________________________________________

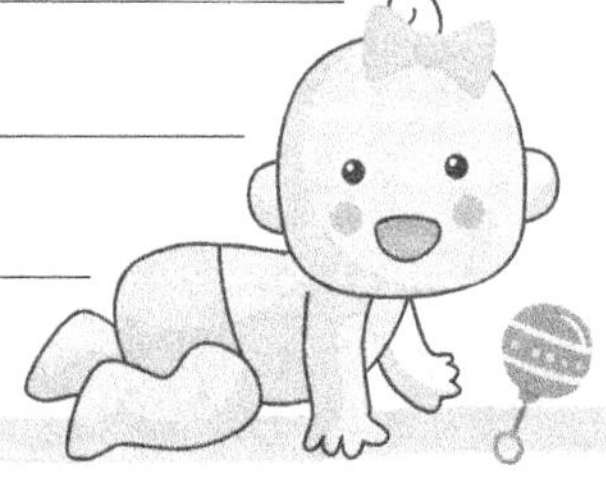

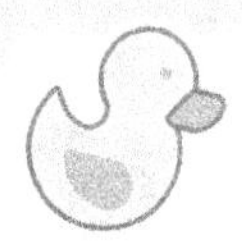

Guest Name

Relationship to Parents

Advice for Parents

Wishes for Baby

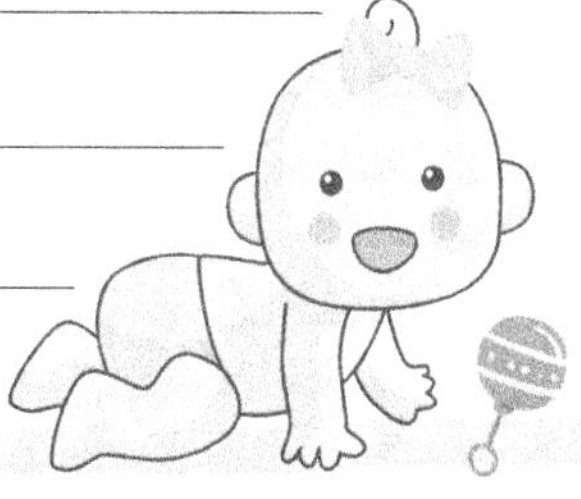

Guest Name

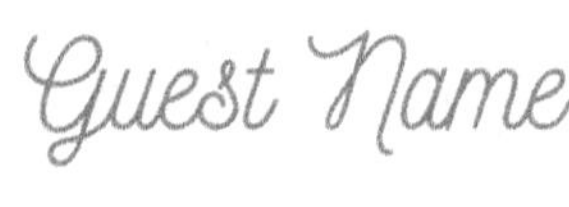

Relationship to Parents

Advice for Parents

Wishes for Baby

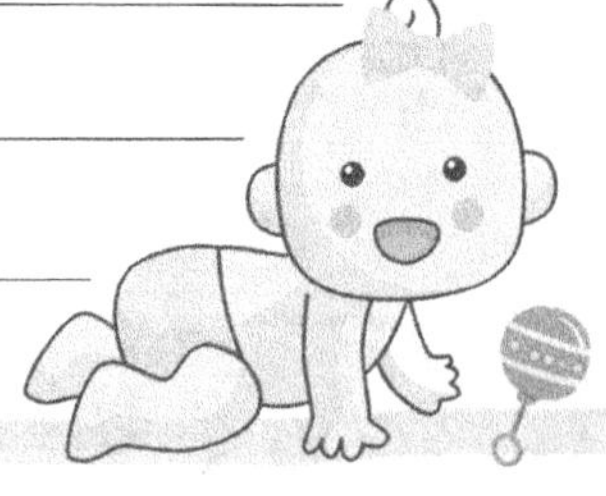

Guest Name

Relationship to Parents

Advice for Parents

Wishes for Baby

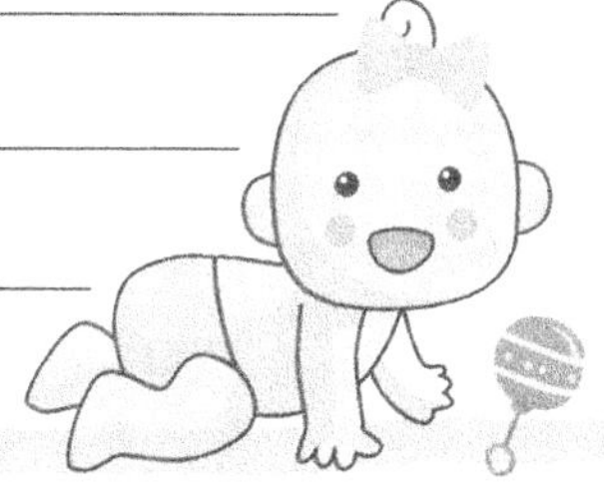

Guest Name

Relationship to Parents

Advice for Parents

Wishes for Baby

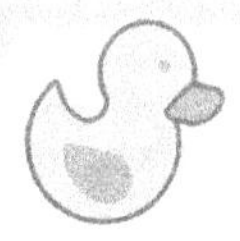

Guest Name

Relationship to Parents

Advice for Parents

Wishes for Baby

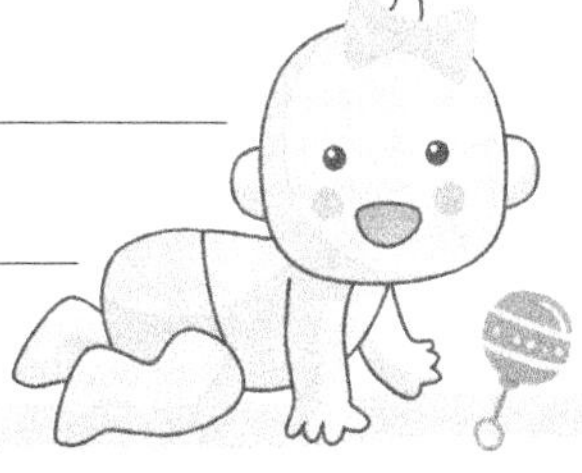

Guest Name

Relationship to Parents

Advice for Parents

Wishes for Baby

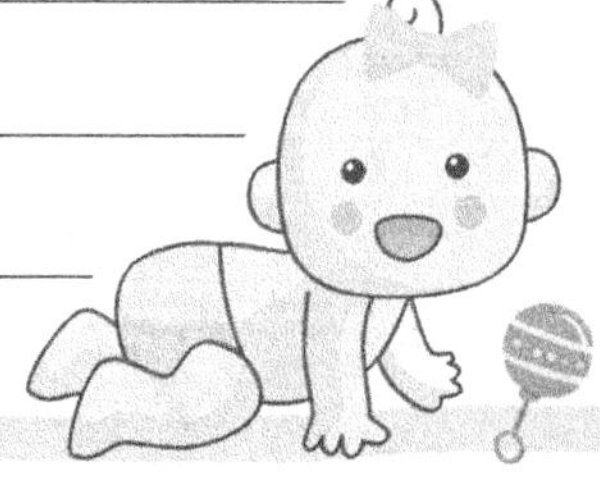

Guest Name

Relationship to Parents

Advice for Parents

Wishes for Baby

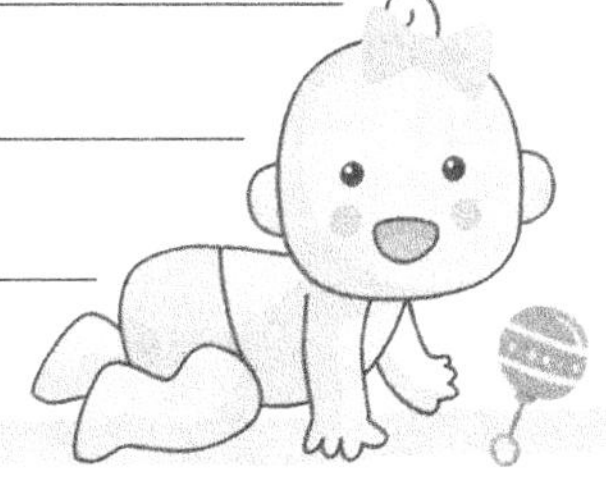

Guest Name

Relationship to Parents

Advice for Parents

Wishes for Baby

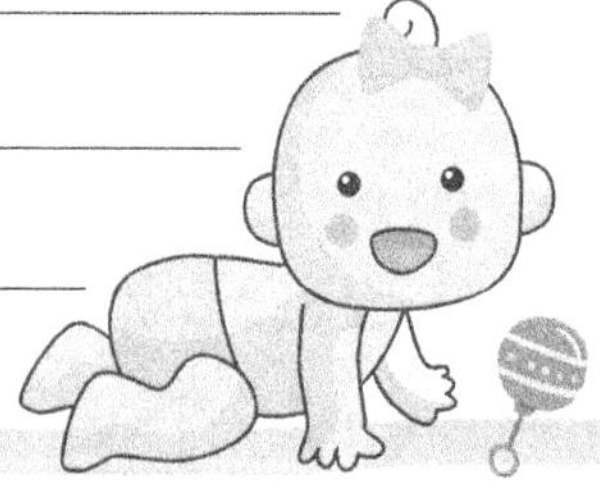

Guest Name

Relationship to Parents

Advice for Parents

Wishes for Baby

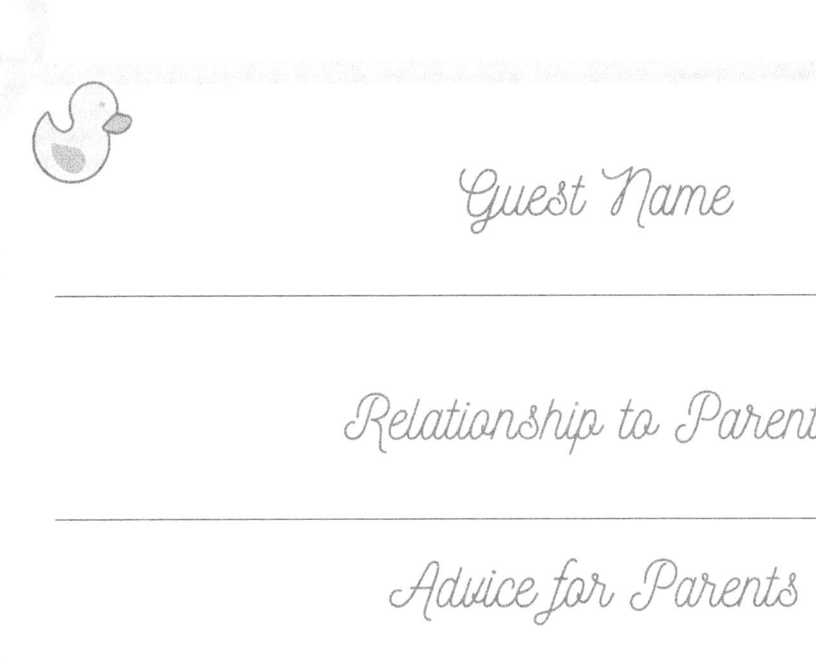

Guest Name

Relationship to Parents

Advice for Parents

Wishes for Baby

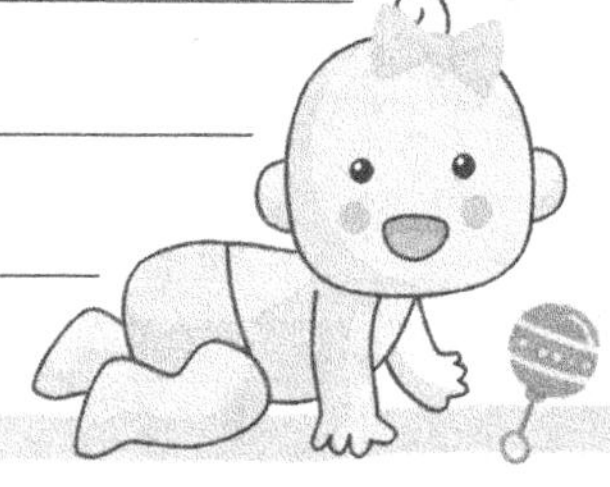

Guest Name

Relationship to Parents

Advice for Parents

Wishes for Baby

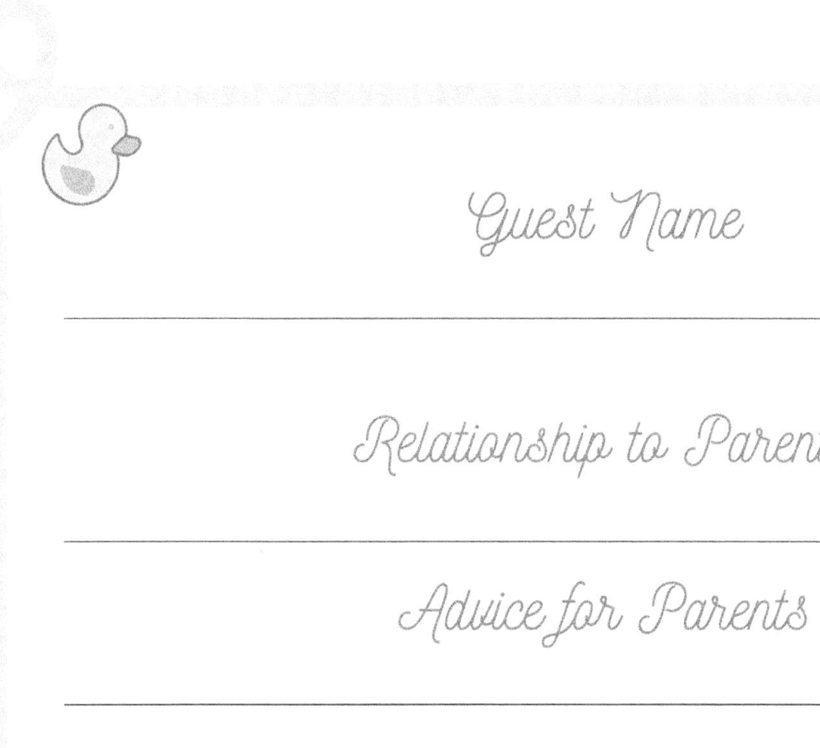

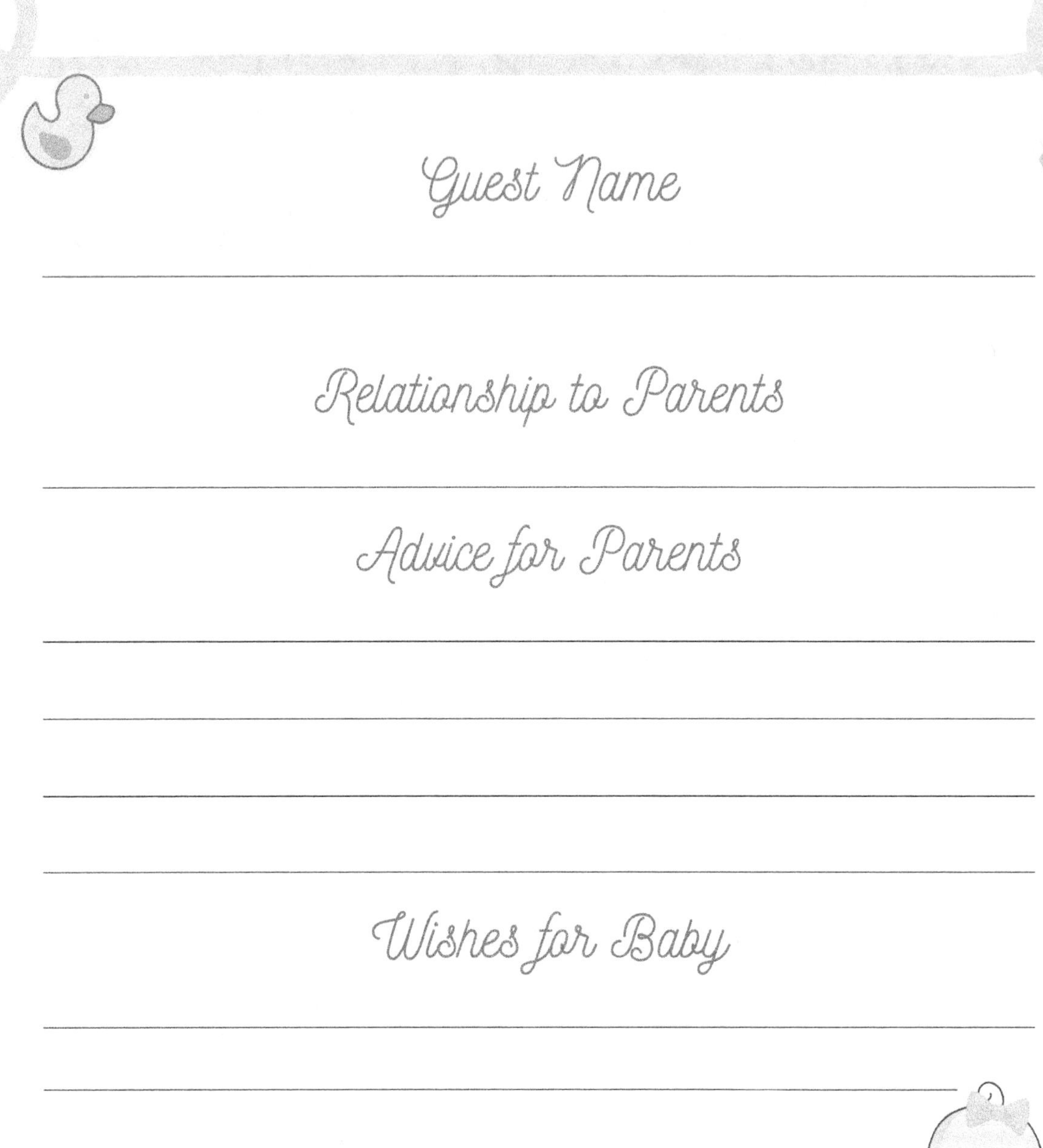

Guest Name

Relationship to Parents

Advice for Parents

Wishes for Baby

Guest Name

Relationship to Parents

Advice for Parents

Wishes for Baby

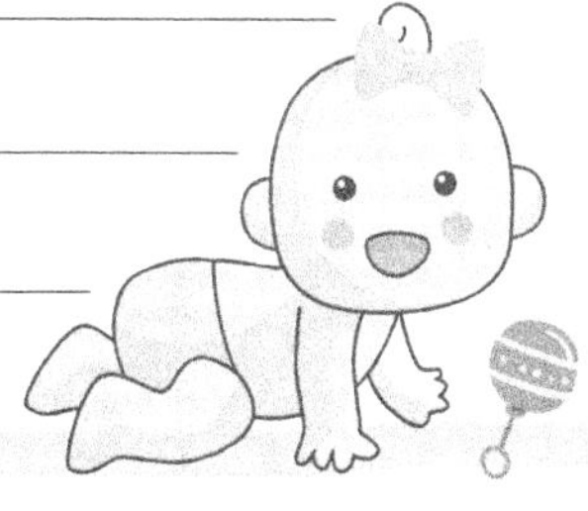

Guest Name

Relationship to Parents

Advice for Parents

Wishes for Baby

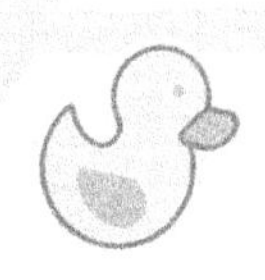

Guest Name

Relationship to Parents

Advice for Parents

Wishes for Baby

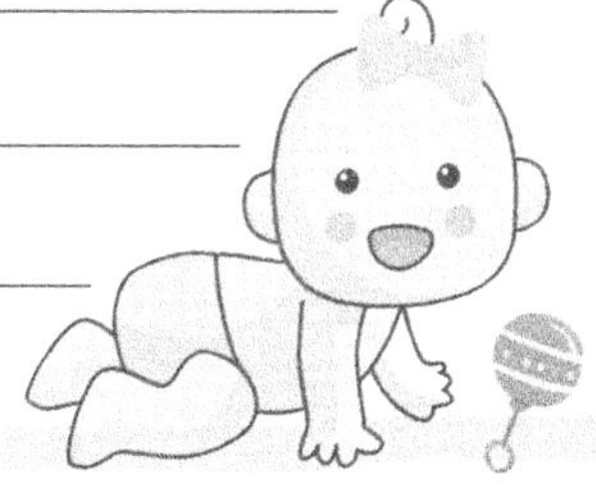

Guest Name

Relationship to Parents

Advice for Parents

Wishes for Baby

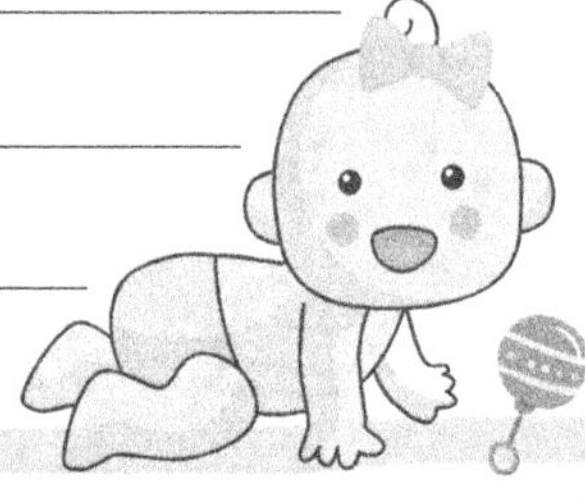

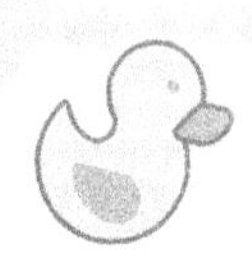

Guest Name

_______________________________

Relationship to Parents

_______________________________

Advice for Parents

_______________________________

_______________________________

_______________________________

Wishes for Baby

_______________________________

_______________________________

_______________________________

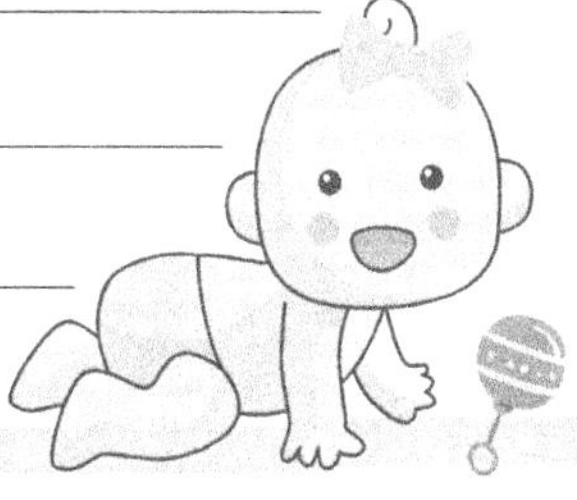

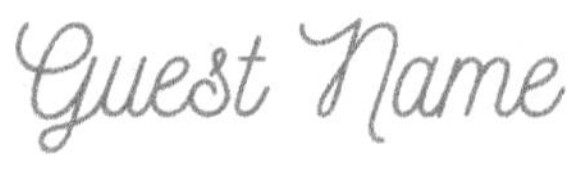

Guest Name

_______________________________________________

Relationship to Parents

_______________________________________________

Advice for Parents

_______________________________________________

_______________________________________________

_______________________________________________

_______________________________________________

Wishes for Baby

_______________________________________________

_______________________________________________

_______________________________________________

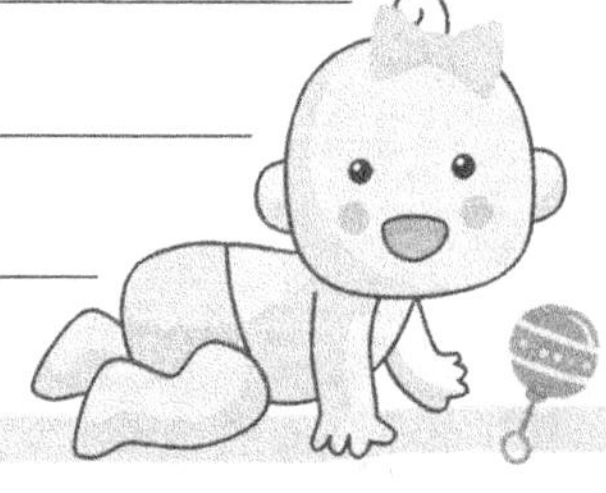

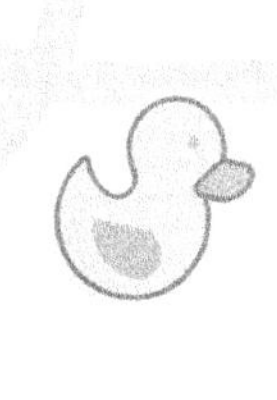

Guest Name

_______________________________

Relationship to Parents

_______________________________

Advice for Parents

_______________________________

_______________________________

_______________________________

Wishes for Baby

_______________________________

_______________________________

_______________________________

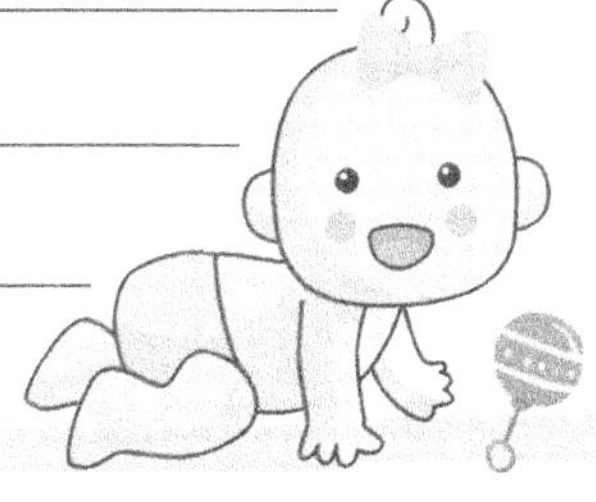

Guest Name

_______________________________

Relationship to Parents

_______________________________

Advice for Parents

_______________________________

_______________________________

_______________________________

Wishes for Baby

_______________________________

_______________________________

_______________________________

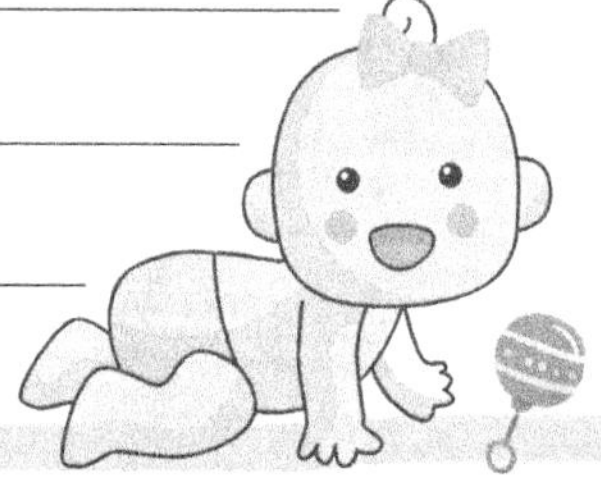

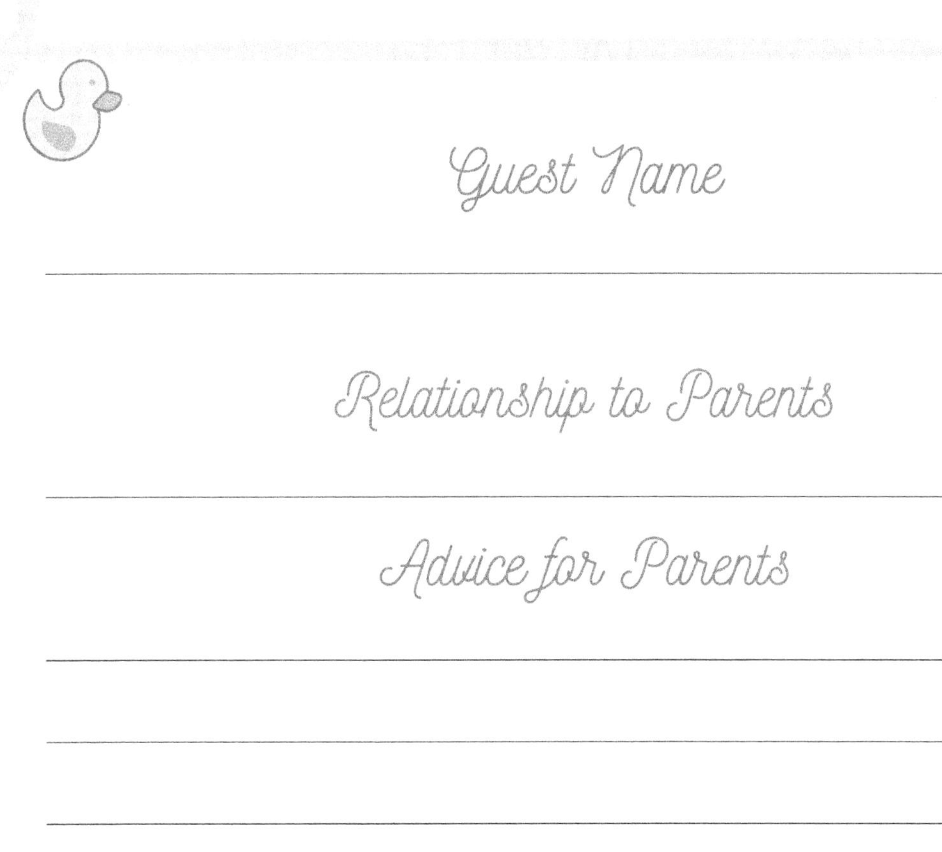
Guest Name

Relationship to Parents

Advice for Parents

Wishes for Baby

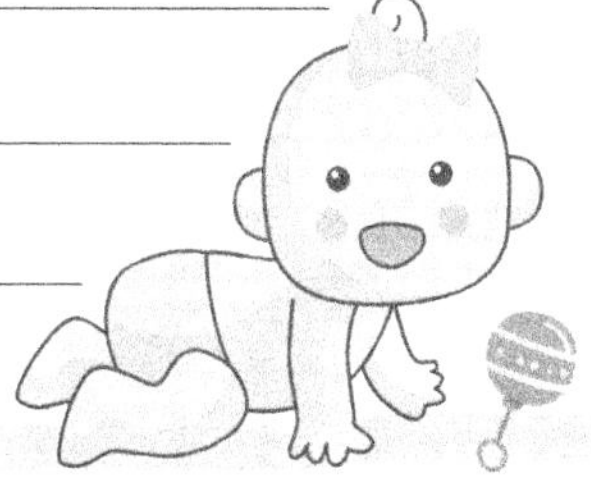

Guest Name

Relationship to Parents

Advice for Parents

Wishes for Baby

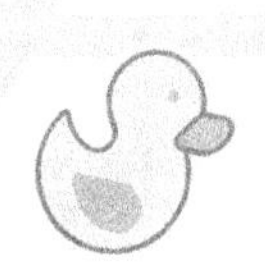

Guest Name

Relationship to Parents

Advice for Parents

Wishes for Baby

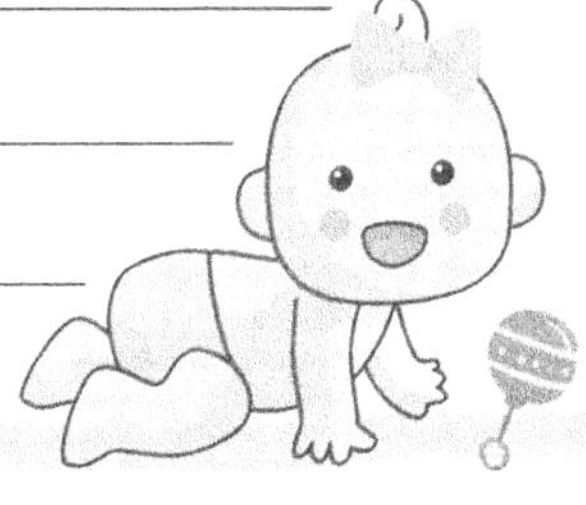

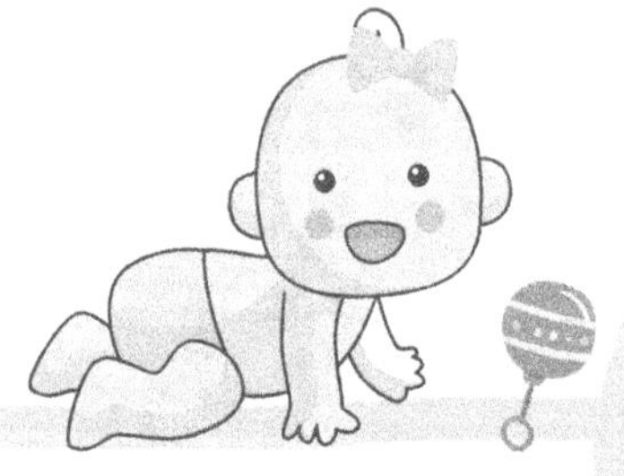

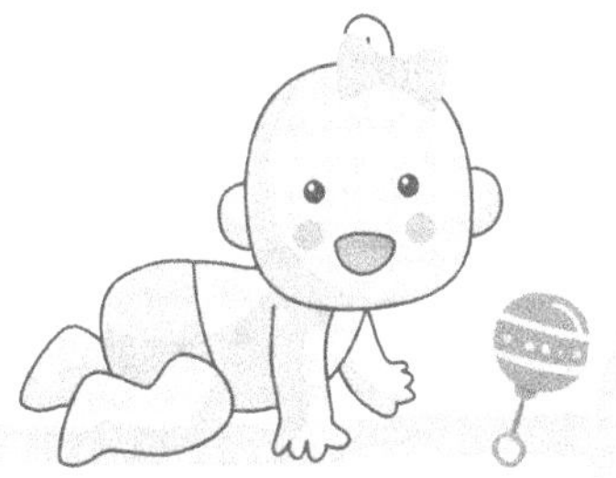

# Notes / Photos

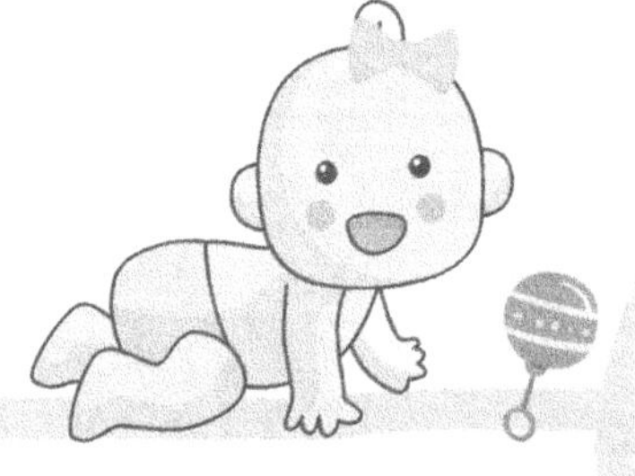

# Notes / Photos

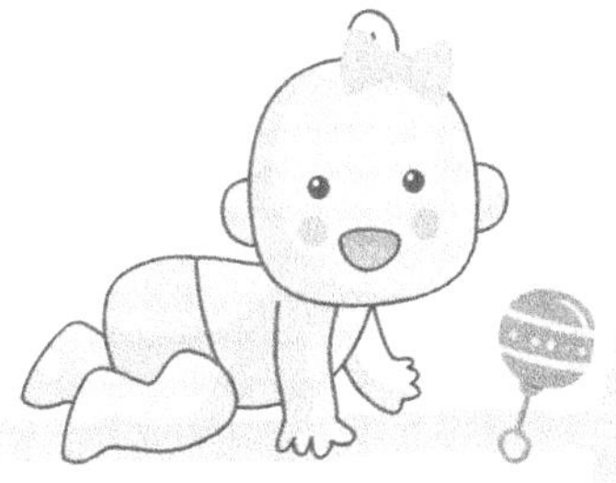

# Notes / Photos

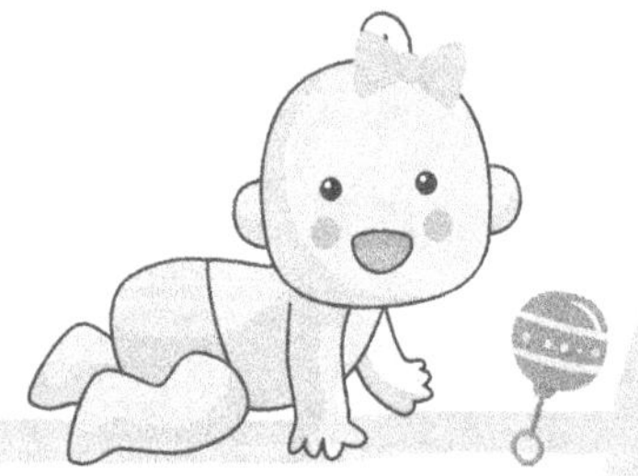

# Notes / Photos

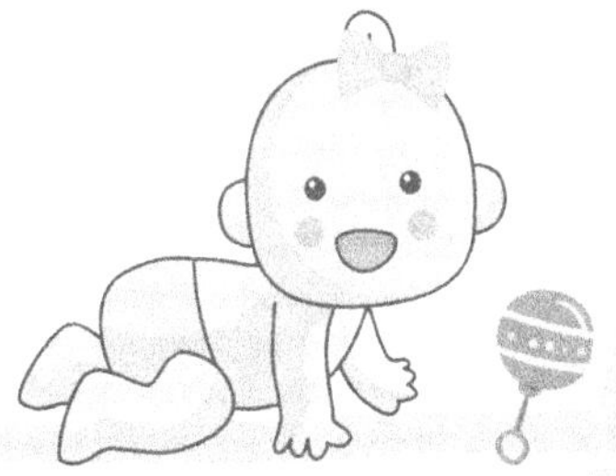

# Notes / Photos

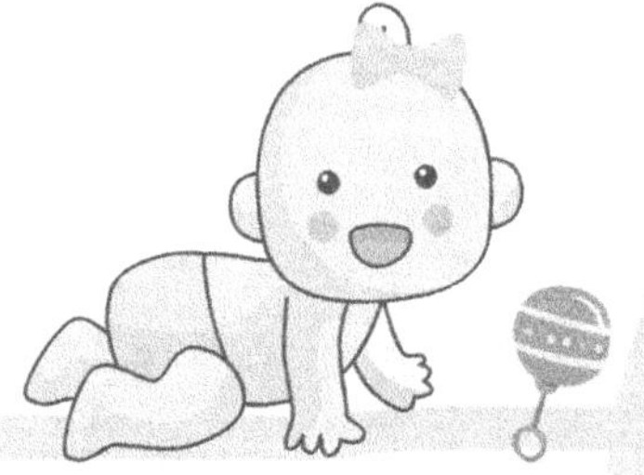

# Notes / Photos

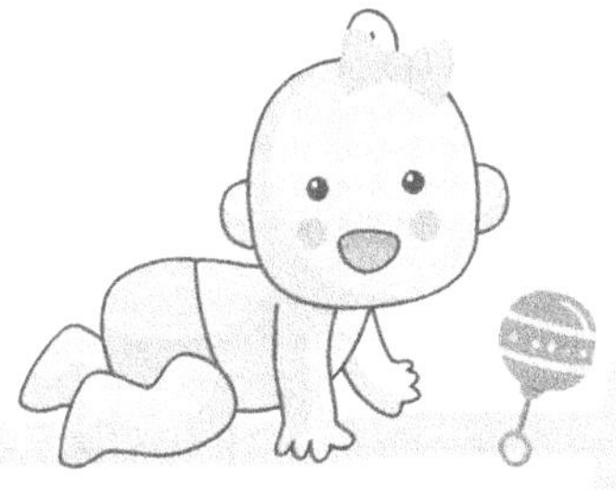

# Notes / Photos

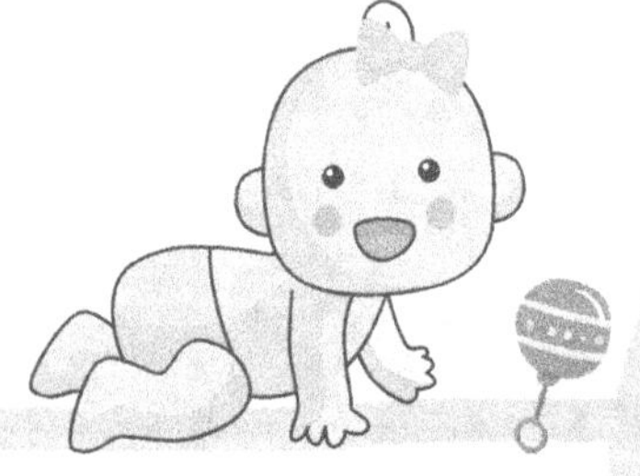

# Gift Log

Name/Email/Phone     Gift

# Gift Log

Name/Email/Phone                    Gift

# Gift Log

Name/Email/Phone      Gift

# Gift Log

Name/Email/Phone                                          Gift

# Gift Log

Name/Email/Phone                    Gift

# Gift Log

*Name/Email/Phone*

*Gift*

# Gift Log

Name/Email/Phone                    Gift

# Gift Log

Name/Email/Phone                    Gift

# Gift Log

Name/Email/Phone          Gift

# Gift Log

Name/Email/Phone                              Gift